the *NEW!* Abs Diet

The 6-Week Plan to Flatten Your Stomach
and Keep You Lean for Life

DAVID ZINCZENKO

EDITOR-IN-CHIEF of Men'sHealth

With Ted Spiker

Some portions of this book have appeared previously
in *Men's Health* magazine.

Illustrations by L-Dopa

Book design by Joe Heroun and Courtney Eltringham,
with George Karabotsos, design director, *Men's Health* Books
and *Women's Health* Books

Library of Congress Cataloging-in-Publication Data is on file with the publisher.

ISBN-13 978–1-60529-276-2 direct-mail hardcover
ISBN-13 978–1-60529-316-5 trade hardcover

Distributed to the trade by Macmillan

2 4 6 8 10 9 7 5 3 1   direct-mail hardcover
2 4 6 8 10 9 7 5 3 1   trade hardcover

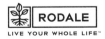

*For every American who has
taken up arms in the battle against obesity.
Today we begin winning the fight...*

CONTENTS

ACKNOWLEDGMENTS

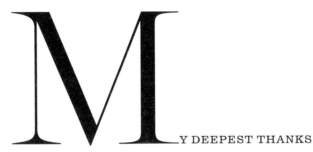

Y DEEPEST THANKS to the extraordinarily talented, hardworking, and dedicated people who have supported me, encouraged me, and inspired me. In particular:

The Rodale family, without whom the Abs Diet series of books would not have been possible.

Jeremy Katz, the original editor of this book, and Ted Spiker, the original co-author.

Jeff Csatari, who helped me revise and update *The New Abs Diet*.

Steve Perrine, the wisest consigliere any boss could ever have.

The entire *Men's Health* editorial staff—the smartest and hardest-working group of writers, editors, researchers, designers, and photo directors in the industry. In the future, when people talk about the glory days of men's magazine publishing, they will be talking about you.

My brother, Eric, whose relentless teasing shamed me into taking better care of myself.

My mother, Janice, who raised the two of us nearly single-handedly. Your strength and kindness guide my every action.

To my dad, Bohdan, who left this world way too early. I wish you were still here.

And to my stepmother, Mickey. Thanks for your guidance and support.

INTRODUCTION

YOUR ABS MAY SAVE YOUR LIFE

You Have Abs. Yes, You.
And This Plan Will Help You Find Them

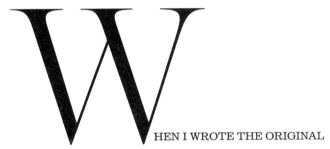

HEN I WROTE THE ORIGINAL
Abs Diet more than 6 years ago, some people thought it was written for beach volleyball players, body-builders, and people who aspire to prance around in front of large-format cameras wearing lace thongs. It couldn't possibly be for real men and women who have more pressing things to do than crunch washboard bellies in a gym all day long.

But then a funny thing happened. It wasn't the athletes or rappers or Victoria's Secret models who picked up the book, but tens of thousands of real men and women. People like you. They gave the program a shot, lost the stubborn pounds, found their hidden abdominal muscles, and, most important, dramatically improved their health.

Then they told their friends about it. And that's how *The Abs Diet* became a *New York Times* bestseller and spawned a half dozen other books, including *The New Abs Diet Cookbook* released in 2010.

I'm proud of the Abs Diet and the impact it has made on people's lives. But I'm not satisfied. Not yet, because so many more people still need to hear the message and learn the secrets to losing weight and firming up their bodies for life. I know that some critics see flat bellies as the modern American symbol of vanity, but dropping pounds, inches, and dress sizes is more than just a way to support the mirror industry. We are at a crucial point in our nation's history: We're too darned fat. Obesity has overtaken smoking as the leading cause of premature heart attacks in the United States. Imagine that—overeating is worse for you than smoking a pack a day. We've forced the smokers out of our restaurants and onto the sidewalk to light up, and yet you can still order an appetizer off the menu that delivers a day's worth of calories and enough grease to turn your colon into a Roman candle. Go figure.

Sixty-seven percent of the population—142 million Americans—are overweight or obese. And a new forecast by University of Chicago researchers estimates that the number of Americans living with diabetes will nearly double in the next 25 years to 44.1 million people.

But it doesn't have to be that way. And I know that the New Abs Diet can help. So, whether you are worried about pre-diabetes or your cholesterol numbers or you just want to flatten your belly in preparation for the approaching beach season, here's my promise: With this book you will improve your health and, yes, find your abs.

As the editor-in-chief of *Men's Health* magazine, and editorial director of *Women's Health*, I know that you—no matter how flabby your belly; how many margaritas you consumed in Cancun; or how many diets you've tried—can develop a flat stomach. See, I analyze health and fitness information with the time and tenacity that you devote to your investment portfolio or fantasy baseball team. It's my job to find the fastest, best, and smartest ways for you to make tremendous gains in your most important investment: your body. And I'm encouraged by all the new research in nutrition and exercise science in the past 6 years, amazing strategies you'll put into practice later in the book. A flat stomach—that is, abs that show—is a worthy goal because it's the ultimate predictor of your health. And you will get there even if you've failed on previous weight-loss attempts and have yo-yoed more than kids at a toy store. I understand your struggle. I've talked to and heard from thousands of people who have shared their weight-loss attempts with me. I know what you've gone through because I, too, know what it's like to feel fat.

As a latchkey kid growing up in the early '80s, I made every mistake in the book. I ate fast food instead of smart food. I played video games when I should've been playing outside. By the time I reached 14, I was carrying 212 pounds of torpid teenage tallow on my 5-foot-10 frame. I wanted to be built like a basketball player, but instead I was built like the basketball. And I paid for it with a steady bombardment of humiliation. My older brother, Eric, would invite friends to our house just to watch me eat lunch. "Don't disturb the big animal," he'd tell his friends. "It's feeding."

Like most kids, I learned my health habits from my parents, particularly my father. He was more than 100 pounds overweight for most of his adult life. Over time, he developed hypertension and diabetes, had a minor heart attack, and would have to stop at the top of a short flight of stairs just to catch his breath. A massive stroke ended his life at 52. My father died because he ignored many signals of failing health—especially the fat that padded his gut.

But I got lucky. When I graduated from high school, I joined the Naval Reserve, where the tenets of fitness were pounded into me, day after day after day. Soon after I graduated from college, I joined *Men's Health* and learned the importance of proper nutrition and—just as important—the danger of carrying around too much fat in your stomach.

Belly fat—the fat that pushes your waist out—is the most dangerous fat on your body. And it's one of the reasons why the Abs Diet emphasizes losing belly fat—because doing so means you'll live longer. Belly fat is classified as visceral fat; that means it is located behind your abdominal wall and surrounds your internal organs. Because it carries an express-lane pass to your heart and other important organs, visceral fat is the fat that can kill you. Just consider one University of Alabama-Birmingham study in which researchers used seven different measurements to determine a person's risks of cardiovascular disease. They concluded that the amount of visceral fat the subjects carried was the single best predictor of heart disease risk.

Whether you want to change your body to improve your health, your looks, your energy levels, or your sex appeal, the New Abs Diet offers you a simple promise: If you follow this plan, you will transform your body so that you can accomplish each and every one of those goals. As a bonus, the New Abs Diet will do something more than just enhance your life; the New Abs Diet is going to save it.

When you think of all you have to gain with the New Abs Diet, it becomes apparent what's wrong with most diet plans out there: They're all about losing. When you consider America's obesity epidemic, losing weight is an admirable goal. But I think there's a fundamental psychological reason why many of these diets fail: There's no motivation in losing. Americans don't like to lose. We don't like to lose board games. We don't like to lose in the market. We don't like to lose our smooth skin, our teeth, or our bodies' fight against gravity. We don't like to lose anything. In a way, we don't even like losing weight because we've all been force-fed the notion that bigger is better. Instead, we're programmed to gain. We want to gain fitness. We want to gain strength. We want to add to our life, not subtract from it. We want to win—and see our results. So consider the New Abs Diet a shift in the way you think about your body and about weight loss. This program concentrates on what you can gain and how you can gain it. As a result of what you'll gain from this program—abs, muscle tone, energy, better health, a great sex life (more on that later)—you'll effortlessly strip away fat from your body and change your body shape forever.

No diet plan would work without good nutrition, so that, of course, is the major focus of the New Abs Diet. You'll not only learn what to eat; you'll learn how to eat to make your body burn fat furiously, as well as how to make sure that you can control the cravings that threaten to add girth to your middle. The focus of the plan revolves around—but does not restrict you to—12 "power-foods" that are among the best sources of protein, fiber, and all the other ingredients and nutrients that help fight fat. When you build your diet around these foods, you will build a new body in the process. But we've taken this weight-loss plan to a whole other level. While nutrition remains a principal component of most diets, too many programs out there focus solely on how to change your eating habits—cut carbs, add cabbage soup, eat at Subway twice a day. Those programs fail to recognize a crucial component of weight control: the fact that our bodies have their own natural fat-burning mechanism . . .

Muscle.

BUILDING JUST A FEW POUNDS of muscle in your body is the physiological equivalent of kicking fat out on its butt and telling it to never come back again. Muscle—in the form of lean muscle mass, not bulky, bodybuilder muscle mass—exponentially speeds up the fat-busting process: One pound of muscle requires your body to burn up to 50 extra calories a day just to maintain that muscle. Now think about what happens if you add just a few pounds of toned muscle in the course of a diet program. It'll take your body up to several hundred extra calories a day just to feed that muscle; essentially, you'll burn off an extra pound of fat every few weeks without doing a thing (and that's not even including the gains you can make by changing your diet). When you combine exercise with the foods that most promote lean muscle growth, the ones that keep you full, and the ones that give your body a well-balanced supply of nutrients, you'll be in the sweet spot, doing what this plan is all about.

You'll change the shape of your body by stripping away your fat and showing off your lean muscle.

Does that mean the New Abs Diet is going to make you burly, muscle-bound, or governor of California? Not at all. The New Abs Diet and the accompanying New Abs Diet Workout emphasize leanness and muscle tone.

Going back to that important investment, you can think about muscle as your compound interest. If you've ever taken a basic economics course, then you understand how compound interest works: If you invest $100 in a high-yield fund and add a little more every month, over time that investment will grow and grow to half a million dollars or more. But you'll have invested only a fraction of the money yourself. Compound interest is what allows you to make the most dramatic financial gains. It's the same concept with your body. Invest in a little additional muscle in the next 6 weeks—through eating the right foods and following a muscle-adding, fat-burning exercise plan—and you'll have invested in a lean and strong body that can last a lifetime because your new muscle will continually break down fat to stay alive.

I'm passionate about this plan because I know it works. I've seen it work, and so will you. During the course of this 6-week plan, you can lose up to 20 pounds of fat (much of it in the first couple of weeks, and from your belly first) and gain several pounds of lean muscle. But the biggest thing you'll notice is that you'll have significantly changed the shape of your body. Some of you will have even more dramatic results (see page 30 for the story of Bill Stanton, who lost 30 pounds in the first 6 weeks on the diet and cut his body fat percentage from 30 percent to 15 percent). The New Abs Diet includes all three components to a successful body-transforming program: nutrition, exercise, and the motivational principles to follow through. I've designed this program to make it easy to stick to, even if you've tried and failed with diets in the past. It's easy to follow because:

▶ Every component of the diet and exercise plan is quick, simple, and flexible enough so that you can easily work it into your life.

▶ Every goal is attainable.

▶ Every principle is supported by well-respected scientific research.

|||||||||||||||||||||||||||||||||||||||||||||||||||||||||||||||||||||||||||||||||||||||||||||||||||||||||||||||||

Foreword: *Diet* Is a Four-Letter Word

In all honesty, I hated to even call this book a "diet" book. That's because the word *diet* has been twisted around to mean something you follow temporarily—you "go on a diet." But if you "go on" a diet, you eventually have to "go off" it. And that's why most diets are really, really bad for you.

Most diets are about eating less food or about restricting you to certain kinds of food. Most of them work in the short term because if you reduce your calorie intake, your body starts to burn itself off in order to keep itself alive. Presto, you lose weight. But here's the problem: The first thing your body does when it's short of calories is to dump the body tissue that takes the most calories to maintain.

That's muscle. So on a low-calorie diet, your body burns away muscle and tries to store fat. Sure, you'll lose weight, and you'll eventually start losing fat as well. But when you "go off" your diet, you'll start to put weight back on. And guess what kind of weight you'll gain? Pure fat. Because you've taught your body a harsh lesson: It has to be on the lookout for potential low-calorie periods in the future, so it had better store fat just in case. You've also used up valuable calorie-burning muscle, so you're likely to end up fatter than you were before your diet. That's why people who try diet after diet not only don't lose weight but also gain it.

The Abs Diet isn't a shotgun, irresponsible approach to weight management. Oh, you'll lose weight, and you'll lose it fast. But you'll lose fat, not muscle. And you'll keep that weight off for life. You'll follow the tenets of the Abs Diet for life, too, because it's about eating lots and lots of great food in smart ways. So enjoy the New Abs Diet. But let's keep that little four-letter word between us, okay?

The New Abs Diet will change the way you think about your body. It's the first plan to count not just the calories your body takes in but the calories your body burns off as well. Using the most cutting-edge nutrition and exercise research, the Abs Diet will show you how to retrain your body to burn fat faster and more efficiently—even while you sleep—and to focus your meals around the foods that inspire your body to keep those calorie-burning fires stoked. The New Abs Diet isn't about counting calories (though you certainly can if that works for you); it's about making your calories count.

Throughout the book, I'll take you through the principles of the New Abs Diet and show you how to follow the 6-week plan. I'll also explain the exercise program (which doesn't have to start until the 3rd week) and give you instructions on how to perform the exercises and how to make the meals. (For the time-crunched, you can cook up many of our powerfood feasts with only a blender.)

To keep you motivated, I've included the stories of real people who credit the Abs Diet with changing their bodies and their lives—not to mention their wardrobes.

THE NEW ABS DIET CHEAT SHEET
(And Portion-Distortion Decoder)

HERE'S AN AT-A-GLANCE guide that summarizes the principles of the New Abs Diet: the 6-week plan to flatten your belly and firm up your body for life. New for this edition, I've added a handy serving-size decoder because I've learned through talking with many veterans of this program that portion control is another useful tool for success with the New Abs Diet.

THE NEW ABS DIET CHEAT SHEET

HABIT	GUIDELINE
EAT	six meals (including snacks) spaced evenly throughout the day.
PLAN	most meals around the **ABS DIET POWER 12** food groups. Each meal should contain at least two of the following:

A lmonds and other nuts
B eans and legumes
S pinach and other green vegetables

D airy (fat-free or low-fat milk, yogurt, cheese)
I nstant oatmeal (unsweetened, unflavored)
E ggs
T urkey and other lean meats

P eanut butter
O live oil
W hole-grain breads and cereals
E xtra-protein (whey) powder
R aspberries and other berries

EMPHASIZE	protein, fiber, calcium, and healthy fats (mono- and polyunsaturated).
LIMIT	refined carbohydrates like baked goods, sugar, white bread, rice and pasta, saturated fats, trans fats, and high-fructose corn syrup.

(chart continues)

1

HABIT	GUIDELINE
DRINK	mostly water. Limit yourself to two or three alcoholic beverages per week to maximize the benefits of the New Abs Diet plan.
CHEAT	once a week by eating anything your heart desires.
EXERCISE	for 20 minutes 3 days a week during weeks 3 through 6 of the program. Exercise is optional for the first 2 weeks, but brisk walking is highly recommended. Total-body strength workouts that can be done at the gym or at home, as well as new interval training programs, are detailed in this book. Two of your strength-training workouts should contain exercises that work your abdominals.

THE PORTION-DISTORTION DECODER

PORTION	ABOUT EQUAL TO...
3 ounces lean meat or poultry	deck of playing cards
3 ounces fish	checkbook
2 tablespoons peanut butter	golf ball
1 tablespoon salad dressing	poker chip
1 ounce hard cheese	3 stacked dice
1 ounce mozzarella cheese	Ping-Pong ball
1 tablespoon butter or mayonnaise	poker chip
1 cup chili or yogurt	baseball
1 serving popcorn	3 baseballs
1 baked potato	computer mouse
1 medium fruit	baseball
1 serving almonds	¼ cup or 12 almonds
1 serving pistachios	¼ cup or 24 pistachios
1 serving sausage	shotgun shell
1 serving (½ cup) ice cream	tennis ball
4 ounces dried spaghetti	diameter of a quarter when held tightly and viewed from end
½ cup cooked spaghetti	tight fist
8 ounces serving of lasagna	2 hockey pucks

Chapter 1

THE NEXT STEP IN WEIGHT LOSS

Cutting-Edge Research Blazes New Paths to a Flat Belly and Healthier Body

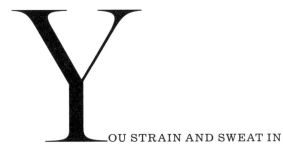OU STRAIN AND SWEAT IN
cardio class, but that belly flab won't budge. Maybe you stepped on the scale
today and were shocked to find that you're heavier than you were two days ago
despite a week of eating every conceivable variation of soy and celery.

What gives? My guess is you've been going about weight loss the wrong
way. But don't beat yourself up; it's not your fault. You've been conditioned to
fight your body's natural fat burners through diets of denial that leave you
coveting your co-worker's meatball sandwich. You've been disappointed by
the workout-of-the-stars du jour, which leaves you feeling sore and frustrated.
You've been misled into thinking that there's some magic bullet out there
that's going to finally give you the body you want, if only you could put up with
the sacrifice and torture for a few weeks.

I have an option for you that's not so painful: take your cues from people who make it their life's work to study weight loss, nutrition, and fitness.
The New Abs Diet is based on the latest scientific study at research hospitals
and human performance labs. In the 6 years since we first published the Abs

Diet books, much more research has been done that further supports its core principles and suggests ways to make it even more effective.

Let's review some of the amazing breakthroughs in nutrition and exercise science that, as you will see, dovetail very nicely with the core tenets of the Abs Diet fitness and weight-loss program. I guarantee they will open your eyes and motivate you to start living the New Abs Diet lifestyle today.

|||||||||||||||||||||||||||||||||||||||||||||||||||||||||||||||||||||||||||||||||||||||||||||||||||||||||||||||||||||||||||||||

Big Numbers

Overweight people are:

- ▶ 50 percent more likely to develop heart disease (obese: up to 100 percent)
- ▶ Up to 360 percent more likely to develop diabetes (obese: up to 1,020 percent)
- ▶ 16 percent more likely to die of a first heart attack (obese: 49 percent)
- ▶ Roughly 50 percent more likely to have total cholesterol above 250 (obese: up to 122 percent)
- ▶ 14 percent less attractive to the opposite sex (obese: 43 percent)
- ▶ Likely to spend 37 percent more a year at the pharmacy (obese: 105 percent)
- ▶ Likely to stay 19 percent longer in the hospital (obese: 49 percent)
- ▶ 20 percent more likely to have asthma (obese: 50 percent)
- ▶ Up to 31 percent more likely to die of any cause (obese: 62 percent)
- ▶ 19 percent more likely to die in a car crash (obese: 37 percent)
- ▶ 120 percent more likely to develop stomach cancer (obese: 330 percent)
- ▶ Up to 90 percent more likely to develop gallstones (obese: up to 150 percent)
- ▶ 590 percent more likely to develop esophageal cancer (obese: 1,520 percent)
- ▶ 35 percent more likely to develop kidney cancer (obese: 70 percent)
- ▶ 14 percent more likely to have osteoarthritis (obese: 34 percent)
- ▶ 70 percent more likely to develop high blood pressure (obese: up to 170 percent)

What You Eat NOW Has a Profound Effect on What You'll Eat LATER

▶ Scientists at the USDA Human Nutrition Research Center at Tufts University found that eating foods that elevate your blood sugar trigger intense cravings for carbohydrates later on. In other words, eating a cookie begets eating more cookies and so on. Eating carbohydrates like baked goods and pasta or sugary foods, they say, promotes greater calorie consumption, not just now, but during the rest of the day.

▶ In 2008, the *British Journal of Nutrition* reported that consuming high-quality protein early in the day results in more sustained fullness compared with eating similar meals in the evening.

▶ A similar study at Purdue University found that men on a calorie-restricted diet had their hunger satisfied the longest when they were given extra protein at breakfast.

Certain Foods May Boost Metabolism and Target Belly Fat

As you'll see, the New Abs Diet program encourages you to try to eat protein with every meal and snack. Protein is recommended for several reasons. It fills you up, it digests more slowly than fast-absorbing carbs do, it spurs lean muscle growth, and it even elevates fat burn, as research continues to prove.

▶ A study in the *International Journal of Obesity* determined that eating two eggs in the morning promotes weight loss. In the experiment, overweight subjects ate a 340-calorie breakfast of either two eggs or a single bagel 5 days a week for 8 weeks. Those who ate these inexpensive protein-packed wonders, the study found, lost 65 percent more weight than the bagel eaters, with no effect on their cholesterol or triglyceride levels.

▶ Whole grains work, too. A 2009 study in the *American Journal of Clinical Nutrition* showed that a calorie-controlled diet rich in whole grains trimmed extra fat from the waistline of obese subjects. Study participants who ate all whole grains (in addition to five servings of fruits and vegetables, three servings of low-fat dairy, and two servings of lean meat, fish, or poultry) lost more weight from the abdominal area than another group that ate the same diet, but with all refined grains.

▶ Another new study in the journal *Obesity* finds that people who eat nuts just twice a week are about 30 percent less likely to gain weight than people who rarely eat nuts. Similar research from the City of Home National Medical Center in Duarte, California, determined that study participants who ate a few ounces of almonds every day lost

||||||||||||||||||||||||||||||||||||||||||||||||||||||||||||||||||||||||||||||||||||||||||||||||||||

Six-Pack Secrets

Weigh yourself. Checking the scale can be motivating. In a study of 3,500 people who maintained 60 or more pounds of weight loss for at least a year, researchers from the National Weight Control Registry found that 44 percent weighed themselves every day. Another study in the *American Journal of Preventive Medicine* found that overweight people are six times more likely to lose weigh if they weigh themselves at least once a day.

Eat, then write. People who kept a food diary lost twice as much weight as those who didn't, according to a study of 1,685 overweight or obese adults at Kaiser Permanente Center for Health Research.

Walk to the water fountain. An Australian study showed that workers who sit for more than 6 hours a day were up to 68 percent more likely to be overweight or obese than those who sat less. The take-home advice: Get out of your chair and move around more. If you work on a computer all day, consider raising the screen and keyboard so that you can stand and do your work.

Leave something on your plate. Cleaning your plate makes for large bellies. In a Cornell University survey, researchers found that the heaviest participants said they stopped eating not when they felt full but when they felt they had made a significant dent in what they thought was a normal-sized plate of food.

Chew, chew, chew, chew. Dutch researchers found that people who chewed large bites of food for 3 seconds consumed 52 percent more food before feeling full than those who chewed smaller bites for 9 seconds. Eating slower and talking between swallows also reduces calorie consumption, studies show.

6½ inches from their waists in 24 weeks, 50 percent more than diet-ers who ate the same number of calories without the fiber-rich nuts.

Diet and Exercise Work Better
Than Exercise Alone

▶ A combination order of whole grains and regular exercise adds up to greater belly-fat loss. In a study conducted by researchers at Penn State University, 50 obese subjects were split into two groups. One was instructed to eat whole grains as their only grain choices; the other was told to avoid whole grains. Both groups were encouraged to do moderate exercise. After 12 weeks, the exercisers who ate whole grains lost a significantly larger percentage of belly fat than those who ate refined grains. Furthermore, their levels of C-reactive protein, a warning signal of heart disease and diabetes, had dropped by 38 percent, while the people who avoided whole-grain foods saw no change in their CRP levels.

▶ A 2008 study at the Human Performance Laboratory at the University of Connecticut suggests a similar strategy for triggering the body to burn more fat. In an experiment, two groups of men were instructed to do resistance training while following either a low-carbohydrate or low-fat diet. After 12 weeks, the lifters who reduced their intake of carbohydrates lost an average of 17 pounds of fat, twice as much as the lifters who followed the low-fat plan. What's more, each member of the low-carb group gained about 2 pounds of lean muscle. "Restricting carbohydrates forces your body to burn fat instead of sugar," says study author and assistant professor Jeff Volek, PhD. And doing so will work as effectively for you as it did for the men in this particular study. The eating plan in this book will show you exactly how to reduce consumption of empty carbs and properly fuel your body for a metabolic lift.

▶ Eating a breakfast of slow-burning carbohydrates like oats can significantly improve calorie-burn during exercise, according to a study at the University of Nottingham reported in 2009 in the

Journal of Nutrition. When active people were given a breakfast of low-glycemic index foods 3 hours before embarking on a 60-minute run, the amount of fat they burned during exercise was 55 percent higher than when they ate a high-carb, high-glycemic breakfast. Are you seeing my point?

Protein Is a Dieter's Friend

▶ Recently, British researchers measured the effect of eating a protein-rich snack after a workout versus a high-carbohydrate snack: Those who consumed 43 grams of protein in a low-carb snack burned 21 percent more fat than the subjects who chugged a sugary post-workout drink. Not only do you expend more energy processing protein than carbs, but the amino acids in protein may lower levels of the stress hormone cortisol in your blood, which could boost your metabolic rate, say scientists at Syracuse University.

Food Is Powerful Medicine

▶ Italian researchers found that eating as little as 1 cup of raw vegetables daily can add 2 years to your life. What does raw have to do with it? They say that cooking depletes up to 30 percent of the disease-fighting antioxidants in vegetables. Here's a quick way to get your quota: Fill a ziplock bag with chopped red and green peppers, broccoli and carrots, and toss them into your work bag with a packet of dressing for an easy lunch. The fat in the dressing will boost your body's absorption of certain nutrients.

▶ Green tea may help exercisers burn more belly fat, according to a 2009 study from the American Society of Nutrition. The 12-week study showed that subjects who drank green tea and did 180 minutes of moderately intense exercise per week lost twice as much weight as people who exercised but didn't drink the catechin-rich beverage. The green-tea group also had larger declines in total abdominal fat, subcutaneous abdominal fat, and triglycerides.

▶ When researchers at Loma Linda University tracked the eating habits of 34,000 Seventh-Day Adventists—a population famous for its longevity—they discovered that those who ate nuts (an Abs Diet Powerfood!) 5 days a week tended to outlive those who didn't eat nuts by 3 years. Scientists believe the monounsaturated fats and fiber in the nuts provide a longevity benefit and help keep weight in check.

▶ Research reported in the journal *Phytochemistry* shows that eating elder berries can help people avoid the flu and may even be effective against H1N1. A different study at UCLA suggests that eating broccoli sprouts triggers nasal cells to produce antioxidants, which can fight off allergies.

▶ A new report by Duke University researchers shows that patients who have nonalcoholic fatty liver disease, a problem in which excess blood sugar converts to fat in your liver, can actually reverse their disease by making easy dietary changes. Simply by swapping whole grains and fruits for fast-absorbing sugars and starches, these people were able to lose weight and eliminate visceral fat deposits.

Exercise Is the Best Medicine

▶ The blubber around your organs, known as visceral fat, is more likely than surface fat to cause disease. Now a new study in *Obesity* shows that exercise is crucial for keeping visceral fat off. In the study, people who lost belly weight and exercised 80 minutes a week didn't regain visceral fat after a year. Subjects who stopped working out, but who still kept a healthy weight, had 25 percent more of the dangerous fat.

▶ A 2009 review of studies at Arizona State University examining the effects of exercise on depression found that people who participated in exercise treatment had significantly lower depression scores than clinically depressed people who did not exercise.

▶ Strength training for four days a week for 13 weeks decreased lower back pain in chronic sufferers by nearly 30 percent, according to a recent report given at the annual meeting of the American College of Sports Medicine.

▶ Two other fitness related studies show that regular exercise relieves constipation in people with irritable bowel syndrome and cigarette cravings in ex-smokers. Now, doesn't that make you want to break a sweat?

How You Work Out Is More Important Than How Long You Exercise

NEW RESEARCH DONE in the years since we first published *The Abs Diet* supports the idea that high-intensity workouts are the most effective at reducing belly fat.

▶ One recent study at the University of Arkansas demonstrated that exercisers who did shorter, high-intensity workouts had a 20 percent reduction in dangerous visceral (deep abdominal) fat after 3 months compared to no change in people who did longer workouts at moderate pace. Researchers say that alternating short bursts of fast walking with slower segments can burn an average of 25 percent more calories.

▶ A Penn State University study found that people who lifted weights while following a program of diet and aerobic exercise had the same weight loss as those who only dieted (or who dieted and performed aerobic exercise). The difference? The lifters lost 5 pounds more fat because almost none of their weight loss came from muscle.

▶ In a 2009 study at the University of Oklahoma, exercise physiologists put a group of people on a resistance-training program that consisted of three workouts a week for 14 weeks. At the end of the study, the participants experienced significant improvements in weight loss and a reduction in waist circumference. The most significant change, however, was in fasting insulin levels, which decreased dramatically.

▶ Another new study demonstrated the belly-fat-frying benefit of adding weight training to a vigorous walking or jogging routine. In the 12-week experiment at Skidmore College, exercisers who did a high-intensity total-body resistance workout along with cardio lost four times as much belly fat when compared with exercisers who only did cardio workouts. The researchers attribute the extra fat loss to two things: the stepped-up calorie burn you get immediately after lifting weights and later, when you increase your lean muscle mass. Whenever you lose weight, it typically comes from both fat and muscle tissue. Resistance training helps you maintain muscle, which prevents a slowdown in your metabolism. A 2009 study from The College of New Jersey offers further support: Participants who performed an intense weight workout before riding a stationary bike burned more fat during the cardio session than other subjects who pedaled but skipped the weight workout. TCNJ researchers speculate that weight training triggers the release of hormones that burn fat.

Why It's So Important to Lose That Belly

NOW THAT YOU'VE had a glimpse of the new research that's going to help you find your abs, let's learn why abs are so important to a healthy body. We'll begin with a quick biology review:

The average American is carrying around about 30 billion fat cells. Each of those buggers is filled with greasy substances called lipids. When you pump doughnuts, corn chips, and fried Snickers bars into your system, those fat cells can expand—up to 1,000 times their original size. But a fat cell can get only so big; once it reaches its physical limit, it starts to behave like a long-running sitcom. It creates spin-offs, leaving you with two or more fat cells for the price of one. Only problem: Fat cells have a no-return policy. Once you have a fat cell, you're stuck with it. So as you grow fatter and double the number of fat cells in your body, you also double the difficulty you'll have losing the lipids inside them.

Many of us tend to store fat in our bellies, and that's where the health dangers of excess weight begin. Some of us store it above the belt, while others store it below the belt. In any case, abdominal fat doesn't just sit there and do nothing; it's active. It functions like a separate organ, releasing substances that can be harmful to your body. For instance, it releases free fatty acids that impair your ability to break down the hormone insulin (too much insulin in your system can lead to diabetes). Fat also secretes substances that increase your risk of heart attacks and strokes, as well as the stress hormone cortisol (high levels of cortisol are also associated with diabetes and obesity as well as with high blood pressure). Abdominal fat bears the blame for many health problems because it resides within striking distance of your heart, liver, and other organs—pressing on them, feeding them poisons, and messing with their daily function.

Now take a look at the people with flat stomachs and six-packs. They're the icons of strength and good health. They're lean; they're strong; they look good in clothes; they look good without clothes. A defined midsection, in many ways,

||||||||||||||||||||||||||||||||||||||||||||||||||||||||||||||||||||||||||||||||||||||||||||||||||||||||||||||||

Baby, Baby, Where Did Our Lunch Go?

Your last meal didn't wind up just in your gut. After a meal, your body begins to apportion the calories to nutrient-hungry organs, growing muscles, and, yes, your belly. Michael Jenson, MD, a professor of medicine in the division of endocrinology, diabetes, and metabolism at the Mayo Clinic, calculated this breakdown of how your body processes food.

10 percent to the kidneys. Kidneys work to make sure the blood is balanced with the right amounts of water and nutrients.

5–10 percent to the heart. The heart gets most of its energy from fat, which provides more long-term energy for the hardworking heart than glucose can.

23 percent to the liver, pancreas, spleen, and adrenal glands. After the liver pulls out nutrients, it stores excess calories as glycogen.

25 percent to muscles. Muscles require a constant source of energy just to maintain their mass, so the more muscle you have, the more calories you burn.

10 percent to the brain. Glucose is brain fuel. It can't be stored long term, which is why people often feel faint if they skip a meal.

10 percent to thermogenesis. The simple act of breaking down the food you just ate takes up one-tenth of your calories.

2–3 percent to fat cells. Your fat cells grow and eventually divide as more and more calories are deposited.

10 percent to no one knows where. Your body's a big place, and some calories go unaccounted for.

has defined fitness. But it also defines something else: A flat stomach is the hall-mark of people in control of their bodies and, as such, in control of their health.

While some people may think that working toward a flat belly is shallower than a kiddie pool, there's nothing wrong with striving for a flat stomach or a defined midsection. Of course, defined abs make you look good—and make others feel good about the way you look, too. (In one survey, both men and women rated abs as the sexiest body part.) And for good reason: When you're in great shape, you're telling the world that you're a disciplined, motivated, confident, and healthy person—and hence a desirable partner. And as you've seen above, sometimes a little vanity can be good for your health. Here's more evidence: A Canadian study of more than 8,000 people found that over 13 years, the people with the weakest abdominal muscles had a death rate more than twice as high as those with the strongest midsections. Such research upholds the notion that flat stomachs do more than turn heads at the beach. In fact, your abdominal muscles control more of your body than you may even real-ize—and have just as much substance as show. In short, here are my top seven reasons why flattening your belly is going to make your life better.

Reason 1: A Flat Belly Will Help You Live Longer

STUDY AFTER STUDY shows that the people with the largest waist sizes have the most risk of life-threatening disease. The evidence couldn't be more con-vincing. According to the National Institutes of Health, a waistline larger than 40 inches for men and 35 inches for women signals significant risk of heart dis-ease and diabetes.

Waist size is an accurate measure of health risk because it gives a good indica-tion of the amount of fat a person is carrrying around, especially in the abdominal area. As I mentioned earlier, belly fat, which sits against the organs and secrets harmful substances, is considered an important risk factor for cardiovascular disease, such as stroke and coronary heart disease, and it leads to a reduction in the body's response to insulin, a precursor to the onset of type 2 diabetes. In fact, recent research indicates that half of all people whose waists measure more than 39.37 inches are insulin resistant.

Now the real scary part: Federal health surveys show that, as of 2008, the average American man's waist measures around 40 inches, an increase of 5 inches compared with 40 years ago. In the past four decades, the average American woman's waist size has grown from 30 inches to 37 inches.

Of course, finding your abs doesn't guarantee you a get-out-of-the-hospital-free card, but studies show that by developing a strong abdominal section, you'll reduce body fat and significantly cut the risk factors associated with many diseases, not just heart disease. For example, the incidence of cancer among obese patients is 33 percent higher than among lean ones, according to a Swedish study. The World Health Organization estimates that up to one-third of cancers of the colon, kidney, and digestive tract are caused by being overweight and inactive. And having an excess of belly fat is especially dangerous. See, cancer is caused by mutations that occur in cells as they divide. Fat tissue in your abdomen spurs your body to produce hormones that prompt your cells to divide. More cell division means more opportunities for cell mutations, which means more cancer risk.

As I inferred earlier, a lean waistline also heads off another of our most pressing health problems—diabetes. It is estimated that 23 million Americans now have type 2 diabetes, and one quarter of them don't even know it. In addition, 57 million more Americans may have pre-diabetes. Fat, especially belly fat, bears the blame. There's a misconception that diabetes comes only from eating too much refined sugar, like the kind in chocolate and ice cream. But people develop diabetes after years of eating high-carbohydrate foods that are easily converted into sugar—foods like white bread, pasta, and mashed potatoes. Scarfing down a basket of bread and a bowl of pasta can do the same thing to your body that a carton of ice cream does: flood it with sugar calories. The calories you can't burn are what convert into the fat cells that pad your gut and leave you with a disease that, if untreated, can lead to blindness, heart attacks, strokes, amputation, and death. And that, my friend, can really ruin your day. But you can control a lot of this: A study tracking 1,400 diabetic people for 9 years found that just trying to lose weight could cut diabetes-related death risk by up to 30 percent.

Upper-body obesity is also the most significant risk factor for obstructive sleep apnea, a condition in which the soft tissue in the back of your throat collapses during sleep, blocking your airway. When that happens, your brain signals you to wake up and start breathing again. As you nod off once more, the same thing happens, and it can continue hundreds of times during the night—making you chronically groggy and unable to get the rest your body needs. (You won't remember waking up over and over again; you'll just wonder why 8 hours of sleep left you dragging.) Fat's role is that it can impede muscles that inflate and ventilate the lungs, forcing you to work harder to get enough air. When Australian researchers studied 313 patients with severe obesity, they found that 62 percent of them with a waist circumference of 49 inches or more had a serious sleep disturbance and that 28 perecnt of obese patients with smaller waists (35 to 49 inches) had sleep problems. Being overweight also puts you at risk for a lot of other conditions that rob you of a good night's rest, including gastroesophageal reflux and asthma. A 3-year French study of 67,229 women found that being overweight doubled the risk of asthma. When Dutch researchers studied nearly 6,000 men, they found that those whose waistlines measured 37 to 40 inches had a significantly increased risk of respiratory problems, such as wheezing, chronic coughing, and shortness of breath. All of this can create an ugly cycle: Abdominal fat leads to poor sleep. Poor sleep means you drag through your day. Sluggish and tired, your body craves some quick energy, so you snack on some high-calorie junk food. That extra junk food leads to more abdominal fat, which leads to . . . well, you get the picture.

I could fill this whole book with evidence, but I'm going to boil it down to one sentence: A smaller waist equals fewer health risks.

Reason 2: A Flat Belly Will Improve Your Sex Life

WOMEN CLAIM THE greatest sex organ is the brain; men say it's approximately 3 feet due south. So let's say we split the geographic difference and focus on what's really central to a good sex life.

You know the old phrase "It's not the size of the ship; it's the motion of the ocean"? Well, take that to heart. We can't improve upon what God gave you (though the New Abs Diet may actually somewhat increase the size of a guy's manhood—more on that in a bit), but we can rebuild your body to maximize the rocking and rolling that goes on below decks. Consider how the following side benefits can help you pull that ship into harbor.

Increased stamina. The thrusting power you generate during sex doesn't come from your legs, it comes from your core. Strong abdominal and lower-back muscles give you stamina and strength to try new positions (or stay steady in old ones), so that sex is as pleasurable as it should be. But even more important, a smaller waistline means that you will be better equipped in another important area—bloodflow.

Better erections, guys. It's no secret that upward of 30 million American men have some kind of erectile dysfunction. Though many things can cause it, one of the major causes is purely a matter of traffic control. Artery-clogging cheeseburgers don't discriminate, so when you're overweight, the gunk that gums up the blood vessels leading to your heart and brain also gums up the vessels that lead to your genitals. Plaque forms on the inside of your arteries, narrowing the passageways that blood must follow. Think of 12 lanes of traffic bottlenecking into one. Your blood vessels can become so clogged in your pelvic area that a sufficient supply of blood can't get through to form an erection. You don't need to have aced calculus to understand this equation: Increased fat equals decreased bloodflow. Decreased bloodflow equals softer (or no) erections. Softer (or no) erections equals "This stinks" squared. (By the way, clogged blood vessels have the same effect on women, leading to decreased lubrication, sensitivity, and sexual pleasure.)

ABS DIET SUCCESS STORY

"I Lost 25 Pounds in 6 Weeks!"

Name: Paul McComb

Age: 28

Height: 5'9"

Starting weight: 180

Six weeks later: 155

Once Paul McComb left college and gained some weight, he figured that extra heft was his to keep for life. But when he walked into a nutrition store and stepped on a scale that told him how much he weighed (180 pounds) and how much he should weigh (155 pounds), something changed: his attitude.

So McComb went on the Abs Diet—and lost 25 pounds.

He made significant changes by doing such things as eliminating the four or five daily Cokes and skipping the midnight chips. He says the transition was easy because the Abs Diet allowed him to eat plenty—six times a day, in fact. "With the eating

Increased length, gentlemen. When it comes to a man and his privates, fat is his body's side-view mirror: Objects appear smaller than actual size. The length of the average man's penis is about 3 inches flaccid, but tht fatter he is, the smaller he'll look. That's because the fat at the base of a man's abdomen covers up the base of his penis. Losing 15 pounds of fat will add up to a half an inch to the length of a man's member. No, Little Elvis is not technically growing, but decreasing the fat that surrounds it will allow all a guy's got to actually show.

Reason 3: A Flat Belly Will Keep You Safe from Harm

IN SCHOOL, YOU were taught the story of Mrs. O'Leary's cow and how, with one awkward misstep, the lumbering bovine knocked over an oil lamp that started the Great Chicago Fire and burned much of that toddlin' town to the ground. That tragedy happened at a time when most urban housing was still built with wood. Today, such a disaster is unthinkable—and not just because we don't let cows into the living room anymore. It's unthinkable because the

six times a day, I didn't feel like snacking on chips," he reports. "I used to not eat at all during the day; then I'd come home, eat dinner, and have chips in the evening. When I started eating all day, it was like, holy cow, I just wasn't as hungry."

McComb says the key to his success was planning meals around the Abs Diet Powerfoods, so he wasn't tempted by vending machines and snack bars. He'd eat turkey on multigrain bread for lunch, have whole-wheat pasta or chicken for dinner, and snack on peanut butter and chocolate milk. He was happy that he didn't have to count calories, watch carbs, or give up the foods he loves. "Under-standing the powerfoods concept and how these foods work together helped me eat—a lot—and still watch the weight come off."

McComb, who did the Abs Diet Workout at home with 20-pound dumbbells, says he'll always incorporate the principles of the Abs Diet into his lifestyle. "I feel a lot better now. I feel more confident because I set a goal for myself and I actually achieved it. Even my skin is a bit clearer. I find I'm getting better sleep, I'm waking up more rested, and the bags under my eyes are going away. Everything seems to be that much better in my life. I'm sure some of my friends are sick of hearing how much weight I lost."

infrastructure of today's cities is built with steel—steel that stands up to fire, earthquakes, and hurricanes.

Think of your midsection as your body's infrastructure. You don't want a core constructed of dry, brittle wood or straw and mud. You want a midsection made of solid steel, one that will give you a foundation of protection that belly fat never could.

Consider a US Army study that linked powerful abdominal muscles to injury prevention. After giving 120 artillery soldiers the standard army fitness test of situps, pushups, and a 2-mile run, researchers tracked the soldiers' lower-body injuries (such as lower-back pain, Achilles tendinitis and other problems) during a year of field training. The 29 soldiers who cranked out the most situps (73 in 2 minutes) were five times less likely to suffer lower-body injuries than the 31 who barely notched 50. But that's not the most striking element. Those soldiers who performed well in the pushups and the 2-mile run enjoyed no such protection—suggesting that good upper-body strength and cardiovas-

||||||||||||||||||||||||||||||||||||||||||||||||||||||||||||||||||||||||||||||||||||||||||||||||||||||||||

Abs Diet FAQs

How much weight will I lose on the New Abs Diet?

I can't give you a firm number, because people's bodies have more variables than a calculus textbook. I can tell you that some people who have used the Abs Diet have lost 25 pounds in 6 weeks. That doesn't necessarily mean that you will, but it means that you might or that you could. Much of your success depends on so many factors—including your intensity of exercise and your starting weight. But we've seen a lot of people who've lost somewhere between 10 and 15 pounds in the first 6 weeks while also gaining a few pounds of muscle, which helps them keep burning fat after that initial 6-week surge.

What percentage of body fat do you have to get to so that you can see your abs?

Finding your abs might feel as daunting as digging through sand to find a buried treasure. But if you dig diligently enough—and by that I mean burning off that extra, unwanted flab—you will find the treasure. As far as the specific body-fat percentage, it varies. I've seen both men and women with body-fat percentages in the teens with defined stomach muscles. For most men, you need to get to around 10 percent. The good news is that if you're exercising regularly, then at least 80 percent of every pound you lose will be fat.

cular endurance had little effect on keeping bodies sound. It was abdominal strength that offered the critical protection. Unlike any other muscles in your body, a strong core affects the functioning of the entire body. Whether you ski, do yard work, or carry the kids away from the candy aisle, your abs are the most essential muscles for keeping you from injury. The stronger they are, the stronger—and safer—you are.

Reason 4: A Flat Belly Will Strengthen Your Back

I HAD A friend who threw out his back maybe two or three times a year. He always did it in the simplest way—sleeping awkwardly or getting out of a chair too quickly. One time, he pulled it out reaching into the backseat of his car to get something for his young daughter. The pain once stabbed him so badly that he collapsed to the ground while he was standing at a urinal. (Imagine that.) His problem wasn't that he had a bad back; it was that he had weak abs. If he had trained them regularly, he could've kept himself from being one of the millions of people who suffer from back pain every year. And yes, he started the Abs Diet Workout, and within weeks his back pain virtually disappeared.

Because most back pain is related to weak muscles in your trunk, maintaining a strong midsection can help resolve many back issues. The muscles that crisscross your midsection don't function in isolation; they weave through your torso like a spiderweb, even attaching to your spine. When your abdominal muscles are weak, the muscles in your butt (your glutes) and along the backs of your legs (your hamstrings) have to compensate for the work your abs should be doing. The effect, besides promoting bad company morale for the muscles picking up the slack, is that it destabilizes the spine and eventually leads to back pain and strain—or even more serious back problems.

Reason 5: A Flat Belly Will Help You Win

IF YOU RUN, bike, play naked Twister, or do any sport that requires movement, your essential muscle group isn't your legs or arms. It's your core—the muscles in your torso and hips. Developing core strength gives you power to perform. It fortifies the muscles around your whole midsection and trains them to provide the right amount of support when you need it. So if you're weak off the serve, strong abs will improve it. If you also play sports where you run a lot, whether it's tennis or tag, abs can improve your game tremendously. That's because speed is really about accelerating and decelerating. How fast can you go from a stopped position at one baseline to stopping at the other baseline? Your legs don't control that; your abs do. When researchers studied what muscles were the first to engage in these types of sports movements, they found that the abs fired first. The stronger they are, the faster you'll get to the ball.

Reason 6: A Flat Belly Will Limit Your Aches and Pains

As YOU AGE, it's common to experience some joint pain—most likely in your knees, hips, and back (but, hey, we've already shown you how building core strength reduces back pain). Getting older can trigger soreness around your feet and ankles, too. The source of that pain might not be weak joints; it might be weak abs—especially if you do any kind of exercise, from serious tennis playing to walking every morning. When you're doing any type of athletic activity, your abdominal muscles help stabilize your body during start-and-stop movements, like changing direction on the tennis court or in kickboxing class. If you have weak abdominal muscles, your joints absorb all the force from

||||||||||||||||||||||||||||||||||||||||||||||||||||||||||||||||||||||||||||||||||||||||||||||||||||||||||

Lose Weight in Your Sleep

A 2009 study in the *American Journal of Public Health* found that people who get enough sleep to feel rested have healthier diets than those who get insufficient sleep. The researchers say sleep-deprived people exhibit lower levels of leptin (the hormone that suppresses appetite) and higher levels of ghrelin (the hormone that makes you hungry). Try these sleep strategies.

▶ Aim for 7 or more hours of sleep each night. A large study of adults found that people who sleep at least 7 hours have the lowest risk of mortality.

▶ Exercise in the afternoon. It can take 6 hours for your body temperature to cool enough after exercising to promote sleep onset.

▶ Avoid caffeine within 8 hours of bedtime and eating within 2. The National Sleep Foundation says both stimulate your system, making it difficult to both get to sleep and control your weight.

those movements. It's kind of like trampoline physics. Jump in the center, and the mat will absorb your weight and bounce you back in the air. Jump toward the side of the trampoline, where the mat meets the frame, and you'll bust the springs. Your body is sort of like a trampoline, with your abs as the center of the mat and your joints as the supports that hold the mat to the frame. If your abs are strong enough to absorb some shock, you'll function well. If they're not strong enough to help cushion the vibrations, the force puts far more pressure on your joints than they were built to withstand.

Reason 7: A Flat Belly Will Help You Sleep Better

HAVING A BIG belly and a fatty neck can trigger chronic loud snorning and its partner, a sleep disorder called sleep apnea. People who have sleep apnea literally stop breathing for a few seconds to more than a minute sometimes hundreds of times a night, disrupting their slumber. They end up feeling exhausted the next morning. Losing weight can often help remedy the problem so you can get a better night's sleep. Exercise helps, too. Australian researchers found that people who lifted weights three times a week for 8 weeks experienced a 23 percent improvement in their sleep quality. If stress is what's causing restless nights, exercise is one of the best things you can do to stop worries from keeping you up. In one study, Texas A&M University scientists found that the fittest people exhibited lower levels of stress hormones in their bloodstreams than subjects who were least fit.

• • •

These are all great reasons to pursue the New Abs Diet. But the best reason is this: The program is an easy, sacrifice-free plan that will let you eat the foods you want and keep you looking and feeling better day after day. It's designed to help you lose weight in the easiest possible ways: by recalibrating your body's internal fat-burning furnace; by focusing on the foods that trigger your body to start shedding flab; and by rebuilding you into a lean, mean, fat-burning machine.

What the Heck Is . . . High Blood Pressure?

You know high blood pressure is bad, but you probably have a little trouble getting your head around the whole concept of how "blood pressure" works. "Can't we just let a little of the blood out and lower the pressure?" you might wonder. If only it were so easy.

When most people think of blood pressure, they think in terms of a garden hose: Too much pressure and the hose bursts, unless you open the valve. But that model is too simple. It helps instead to think of your circulatory system as more like the Erie Canal—a series of locks and gates that help move blood around to where it's needed. See, gravity works on your blood just like it works on the rest of your body: It wants to pull everything downward. So imagine yourself hopping out of bed tomorrow morning and standing up. Gravity wants to take all that blood that's distributed throughout your body and pull it down into your feet. You, on the other hand, would like that blood to pump to your brain, where it can help you figure out where the hell your keys are.

On cue, arteries in the lower body constrict while the heart dramatically increases output. The instant result: Blood pressure rises, and blood flows to the brain. Ahh, there they are—in the dog's water dish, right where you left them.

It's an ingenious system, but one that's incredibly easy to throw out of whack. When you pack on extra padding around your gut, your heart pumps harder to force blood into all that new fatty tissue. When you nosh on potato chips and other high-sodium foods, your body retains water in order to dilute the excess sodium, increasing overall blood volume. When you line your arteries with plaque from too many fatty meals, pressure increases as the same amount of blood has to squeeze through newly narrowed vessels. When you let the pressures of the day haunt you into the night, your brain pumps out stress hormones that keep your body in a perpetual state of fight-or-flight anxiousness, also forcing your heart to pump harder. High-salt, high-fat diets and an excess of stress all combine to create a dangerous situation.

Much to the dismay of Quentin Tarantino fans, letting out some blood won't relieve the pressure. Your heart is still pumping, and your blood vessels are still dilating and contracting to make sure the blood goes where it's needed. When the pressure remains high for years on end, thin-walled vessels in the brain can burst under extreme pressure; brain cells die as a result in what's known as a hemorrhagic stroke. Or hypertension can cause plaque buildup in one of the brain's arteries, eventually cutting off blood-flow. (High blood pressure damages smooth artery walls, creating anchor points for plaque to latch onto.) Kidney failure or a heart attack can also follow from dangerous plaque accumulations.

Then there's the plain old wear and tear that high blood pressure causes on your ticker. Over time, the extra work brought on by high blood pressure causes the walls of the heart to stiffen and thicken. The heart becomes a less efficient pump, unable to push out as much blood as it takes in. Blood backs up, the heart gives out, and the coroner scribbles "congestive heart failure" on your chart.

Ideally, your blood pressure should be lower than 120/80. What do those numbers mean? The top number, called the *systolic* pressure, is the pressure generated when the heart beats. The bottom number is the *diastolic* pressure, the pressure on your blood vessels when the heart is resting between beats. Higher readings are broken out into three categories:

▶ **Prehypertensive: 120–139 systolic/80–89 diastolic.** Prehypertensives should start worrying about their BP, focusing on diet and exercise tips like those found in this book. You may not see the flashing lights in your mirror right now, but your radar detector just went off. Time to slow down.

▶ **Stage I hypertensive: 140–159 systolic/90–99 diastolic.** For people who fall in this range, drug therapy is usually recommended in addition to lifestyle changes. Your risk of heart attack or stroke is elevated, and you need to be under a doctor's care.

▶ **Stage II hypertensive: 160 or greater systolic/100 or greater diastolic.** Advanced drug therapy is often a must for people at this level, who face a serious risk of being maimed or killed by their condition.

So, two questions: Do you know what your blood pressure is? If not, are you freaked out enough by now to start taking care of it? Fortunately, the Abs Diet Powerfoods can help by cutting down on the bad fats in your diet and increasing the good ones—and by slashing away some of those extra pounds. So can the New Abs Diet Workout, as well as a few stress-reduction techniques. (To find out how you can help manage your stress level, see "How Stress Makes You Fat" on page 163.) In the meantime, try attacking the problem with some of these simple tips:

Cut salt, slice bananas. A study published in a 2009 edition of the the *Archives of Internal Medicine* suggests that a combination of eating more potassium-rich

(continued)

ABS DIET HEALTH BULLETIN

What the Heck Is . . . High Blood Pressure? (cont.)

foods while reducing sodium intake lowered blood pressure more effectively than doing any one of those strategies alone. The study at Loyola University showed that cardiovascular disease increased by 50 percent for participants with a high sodium-to-potassium ratio in their blood. Potassium helps sweep excess sodium from the circulatory system, causing the blood vessels to dilate. Studies show that not getting at least 2,000 milligrams of potassium daily can set you up for high blood pressure. Other good sources of potassium are sweet potatoes, spinach, raisins, papayas, lima beans, and tomatoes.

Make it a low-sodium V8. Make that two 5.5-ounce cans: 11 ounces of V8 contains nearly 1,240 milligrams of potassium. The tomato juice also contains lycopene and lutein, two phytochemicals that have their own blood pressure–lowering properties.

Reduce your consumption of cold cuts. One slice of ham contains 240 milligrams of sodium, more salt than you'll find on the outside of two pretzel rods. The point: Lose the lunchmeat, and lower your blood pressure. A recent study found that prehypertensive people who reduced their daily sodium consumption from 3,300 to 1,500 milligrams knocked nearly 6 points off their systolic blood pressure and close to 3 off their diastolic. If you want to have your hoagie and eat it, too, at least switch to the Boars Head line of low-sodium meats—ham, turkey, roast beef—and leave the pickle on your plate (833 milligrams of sod-ium). Another rule of thumb: If a food comes canned or jarred, it's probably a salt mine.

Go two rounds and out. Make the second drink of the night your last call for alcohol. In a landmark study published in the *New England Journal of Medicine,* researchers found that one or two drinks a day actually decreased blood pressure slightly. Three drinks or more a day, however, elevated blood pressure by an average of 10 points systolic and 4 diastolic. The type of alcohol doesn't matter. Heck, order a screwdriver: Orange juice is one of the best sources of blood pressure–lowering potassium.

Drink more tea. An American Heart Association study found that people who drank 2 cups of tea a day were 25 percent less likely to die of heart disease than those who rarely touched the stuff. The reason: Flavonoids in the tea not only improve blood vessels' ability to relax but also thin the blood, reducing clotting.

Top your toast. Black currant jelly is a good source of quercetin, an antioxidant that Finnish researchers believe may improve heart health by preventing the buildup of the free radicals that can damage arterial walls and allow plaque to penetrate.

Have a Mac(intosh) attack. Men who frequently eat apples have a 20 percent lower risk of developing heart disease than men who eat apples less often.

Eat fresh berries. Raspberries, strawberries, and blueberries are all loaded with salicylic acid—the same heart disease fighter found in aspirin.

Order the tuna. Omega-3 fats in tuna and other fish as well as flaxseed help strengthen heart muscle, lower blood pressure, prevent clotting, and reduce levels of potentially deadly inflammation in the body.

Eat oatmeal, an Abs Diet Powerfood! In two large and long-term studies, people who ate whole-grain foods instead of refined carbs significantly lowered their risk of hypertension.

Squeeze a grapefruit. One grapefruit a day can reduce arterial narrowing by 46 percent, lower your bad cholesterol level by more than 10 percent, and help drop your blood pressure by more than 5 points.

Buy calcium-fortified OJ. Increasing the calcium in your diet can lower your blood pressure. By drinking calcium-enriched orange juice, you'll derive a benefit from the vitamin C as well. According to research from England, people with the most vitamin C in their bloodstreams are 40 percent less likely to die of heart disease.

Snack on pumpkin seeds. One ounce of seeds contains 151 mg of magnesium, more than a third of your recommended daily intake. Magnesium deficiencies have been linked to most risk factors for heart disease, including high blood pressure, elevated cholesterol levels, and increased buildup of plaque in the arteries. Other great sources: halibut (170 milligrams in 7 ounces of fish), brown rice (1 cup, 84 milligrams), chickpeas (1 cup, 79 milligrams), cashews (1 ounce, 74 milligrams), and artichokes (one gives you 72 milligrams).

Change your oil. Researchers in India found that men who replaced the corn and vegetable oils in their kitchens with monounsaturated fats (olive oil or, in this case, sesame seed oil) lowered their blood pressure by more than 30 points in just 60 days without making any other changes in their diets.

Cut down on mindless candy snacking. A compound in licorice root has been shown to spike blood pressure—especially in men who eat a lot of black licorice. Fruit-flavored licorice, however, doesn't contain the compound.

THE NEW ABS DIET START-UP KIT

THIS SIMPLE SHOPPING LIST will give you everything you need to dive right into the New Abs Diet and the New Abs Diet Workout.

BUY ONCE

Blender

Ground flaxseed, 1 pint

Multivitamins, such as Centrum, 1 jar

BASIC SHOPPING LIST—THE ABS DIET POWER 12 AND RELATED FOODS

Almonds, slivered or whole

Beans of choice

Spinach, fresh or frozen

Dairy (fat-free or low-fat milk and vanilla yogurt)

Instant oatmeal (unsweetened, unflavored)

Eggs

Turkey, sliced

Peanut butter, all-natural (no added sugar)

Olive oil

Whole-grain breads and cereals

Extra-protein (whey) powder, vanilla and chocolate, 1-quart containers

Raspberries, fresh and frozen

Plus:

Black beans

Blueberries, frozen

Canned tuna

Cannellini beans

Chicken breast

Craisins (dried, sweetened cranberries)

Garbanzo beans

Grapefruit

Green vegetables of choice

Italian salad greens

Lean ground beef

Long-grain rice

Mixed greens

Pecans

Pine nuts

Roasted cashews and peanuts, unsalted

Shrimp, frozen

Strawberries, fresh or frozen

Trout, smoked salmon, or other lean fish of choice

Whole-wheat pasta

SHOPPING LIST–INGREDIENTS FOR RECIPES
(SEE RECIPES FOR INDIVIDUAL AMOUNTS)

Avocado

Baby carrots

Balsamic and red wine vinegars

Bananas

Barbecue sauce

Basil

Beef jerky

Brown rice

Canadian bacon

Canned chicken stock

Canned mandarin orange slices

Canned peeled tomatoes

Canned pumpkin

Cantaloupe

Carnation Instant Breakfast packets

Cayenne pepper

Celery

Chili powder

Chives

Chocolate syrup

Cilantro

Cinnamon

Corn, frozen

Cornmeal

Cucumber

Curry powder

Dijon mustard

Dried chili mix

Fat-free mayonnaise

Flat bread

Flour

French baguette

French green beans

Fresh ginger

Garlic

Green and red bell peppers

Ground buffalo

Guacamole

Housin sauce

Honey

Honeydew melon

Honey-wheat English muffins

Instant grits

Italian-seasoned bread crumbs

Italian seasoning

Jalapeño peppers

Ketchup

Lean sirloin steak

Lean sliced roast beef

Lemons and limes

Lemon juice concentrate, frozen

Low-fat balsamic vinaigrette, ranch, and Thousand Island salad dressings

Low-fat ice cream (vanilla and butter pecan)

Low-fat Italian salad dressing packet

Maple syrup

Mexican-style tomatoes

Mint, fresh or dried

Mushrooms

Navy beans

Onions, green, red, and white

Onion soup mix

Orange juice

Oranges

Oregano

Paprika

Parsley

Peanut oil

Pork chops, boneless

Portobello mushrooms

Prosciutto

Red pepper flakes

Reduced-fat cheese (American, blue cheese, Cheddar, cottage, cream, feta, mozzarella, ricotta, Swiss)

Raisin bread

Raisins

Red and Granny Smith apples

Reduced-sodium soy sauce

Roasted red peppers

Romaine lettuce

Rosemary

Rye bread

Salsa

Saltine crackers or bread crumbs

Sauerkraut

Spaghetti sauce

Stir-fry sauce

Steel-cut oats

Sweet corn

Tabasco sauce

Tomatoes

Tomato sauce

Tortilla chips

Trans fat–free margarine

Turkey bacon

Turkey sausage

Watermelon

Whole-wheat pitas

Whole-wheat toaster waffles

Whole-wheat tortillas

Worcestershire sauce

FOR AT-HOME EXERCISE

(A GYM SHOULD HAVE ALL NECESSARY EQUIPMENT)

Exercise mat
(optional)

Flat bench
(optional but
recommended)

One or two pairs
of medium-weight
dumbbells (5 to
25 pounds for
someone with some
experience lifting
weights; lighter for
beginners)

Running shoes

Swiss ball (optional
but recommended)

Exercise bands for
resistance training
while traveling or
at home

Chapter 2

EAT THIS, WEIGH LESS
Why the New Abs Diet Works When Other Diets Fail

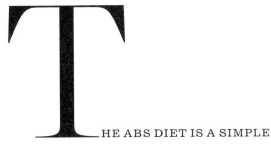

THE ABS DIET IS A SIMPLE plan built around 12 nutrient-packed foods that, when moved to the head of your dietary table, will give you all the vitamins, minerals, and fiber you need for optimum health while triggering lean muscle growth and firing up your body's natural fat burners. (Tell me this isn't a meal plan you can stick to!)

A lmonds and other nuts

B eans and legumes

S pinach and other green vegetables

D airy (fat-free or low-fat milk, yogurt, cheese)

I nstant oatmeal (unsweetened, unflavored)

E ggs

T urkey and other lean meats

P eanut butter

O live oil

W hole-grain breads and cereals

E xtra-protein (whey) powder

R aspberries and other berries

I've chosen these foods both for their nutritional content and their simplicity. That's why I based the Abs Diet on common foods that are easy to prepare and enjoy. The way I see it, most other diet plans are too complicated and invite failure in three major ways.

1. They reduce calories too severely. With a strict—or drastic—calorie reduction, you may lose weight at first, but you're left hungry. When you're hungry, you've increased the chances that you'll gorge at some point during the day. When you gorge, you feel as if you failed, then feel guilty for failing, then drop off the plan and resume your chocolate-for-breakfast habits. With the Abs Diet, however, you'll never go hungry—in fact, you'll find yourself eating much more often than you do now: six times a day!

2. They restrict too many foods. It would be easy to build a plan that didn't include pasta, pizza, or savory bruschetta. But if I did that, you'd ditch the plan the first time you drove past your favorite Italian restaurant. Even though changing your eating habits is a

---

ABS DIET SUCCESS STORY

"I Went from Brando to Rambo!"

Name: Bill Stanton

Age: 40

Height: 5'8"

Starting weight: 220

Six weeks later: 190

Bill Stanton, a security consultant, had been pumping iron since he was 15. But even with his rigorous weight training, he kept getting fatter: By the time he reached 40, he had ballooned to 220 pounds on his 5-foot-8 frame. Why? Because Stanton's diet and exercise routine consisted of doing bench presses and squats and then finishing the night with chicken wings and booze.

"My pants were fitting me like a tourniquet, and it was like I was in a bad marriage—I was living comfortably uncomfortable," Stanton says. "The Abs Diet challenged me to get on the program, step up to the plate, and step away from the plate."

fundamental part of this program, I think there's a greater chance you'll stick to the plan if you don't have to give up everything you like. It's normal to have steaks off the grill, Mom's pie at the holidays, a glass of wine or beer after work. If you deprive yourself of every food that tastes good, there's not much incentive for even the most motivated person to stick to the plan for longer than a few weeks. The Abs Diet is about eating the foods you enjoy—and indulging yourself when need be.

3. They don't take into account lifestyle. If we all had a chef to prepare our meals—or even more than a few minutes to do it ourselves—losing weight would be much simpler. But when was the last time you had 2 hours to prepare a meal? We're all busy. We eat in restaurants. We order in. We hit drive-throughs. We hustle food on the table to satisfy the needs of our families and to save as much energy as possible. Yes, we wish we had time to tally fat-gram totals; measure every ounce of food; or prepare elaborate, good-for-you dishes. But the reality is that most of us won't, no matter how much

---

After following the Abs Diet for 6 weeks, Stanton lost 30 pounds—and has cut his body fat from 30 percent to 15 percent. "I looked pregnant. Now I look like Rambo."

Stanton appreciates the diversity of the Abs Diet meals and the plan's total-body approach to working out, though he admits that eating six times a day took some getting used to. "What I had to do was learn to eat to live, not live to eat," he says. And then, he says, everything just rolled from there. Once his mental approach changed—being committed to the plan, limiting the number of times he partied at night, and eliminating late-night meals—he

was able to turn everything around. "You wake up attacking the day rather than waiting for the day to end," he says.

Now, everything just feels better. He's always in a good mood. He walks taller. He has more energy. And now he's a model for others.

"I work out at Sports Club L.A., where people are *really* focused on looking great," he says. "Even there, guys and girls all come up to me. One guy said, 'You are kicking butt. Everybody sees that transformation. You're inspiring a lot of people.'"

weight we need to lose. We have commitments to jobs and families, and we spend so much time doing everything from commuting to paying the bills and taking care of the kids that a mango-shrimp masterpiece hardly tops the priority list. The Abs Diet is what you need: a low-maintenance program with low-maintenance foods and even lower-maintenance recipes.

For these reasons, many of today's most popular diets offer only short-term weight loss and long-term weight gain.

As I said in the introduction to this book, most diets are about losing—and Americans don't like to be losers. The New Abs Diet is about gaining. The New Abs Diet is based on the simple notion that your body is a living, breathing, calorie-burning machine and that by keeping your body's fat furnace constantly stoked with lots and lots of the right foods—and this is important—at the right time, you can teach it to start burning off your belly in no time. In fact, this diet can help you burn up to 12 pounds of fat—from your belly first—in 2 weeks or less. And just look at what you'll gain in return.

You'll gain meals. Americans have huge appetites. We hunger for success, we hunger for freedom, and yeah, we hunger for food. Traditional calorie- or food-restricting diets run counter to this uniquely American appetite. They leave us hungry, miserable, and one Twinkie away from a total couch collapse. But not the New Abs Diet. You will eat on this program—and eat often. In fact, you'll be refueling constantly, and with every delicious meal or snack, you'll be stoking your body's natural fat burners. Imagine that: Every time you eat, you help your body lose weight and turn flab into abs.

You'll gain some tone. With the New Abs Diet and the New Abs Diet Workout, eating the right foods means you'll be growing more muscle. With added muscle, you'll lose more fat. This program converts the food you eat into muscle. The more lean muscle mass you have, the more energy it takes to fuel it— meaning that calories go toward sustaining your muscles rather than being converted to fat. In fact, research shows that adding lean muscle mass acts as a built-in fat burner. Again, for every pound of muscle you gain, your resting metabolic rate goes up as much as 50 calories a day. The strength-training component can put several pounds of muscle onto your body. You won't beef up like a bodybuilder, but you will build enough muscle to shrink and tighten your belly—and, depending on your starting point, show off your abs. When you add exercise into the mix, you can think of it as a simple equation.

MORE FOOD + MORE MUSCLE = LESS FLAB

Now, consider the alternative.

LESS FOOD + LESS MUSCLE = MORE FLAB

Isn't it incredible that most diets focus on the "less food" equation? And isn't it time we changed that? (Sure, some studies have shown that you'll live longer on a superrestrictive diet of less than 1,400 calories a day. But given how such a plan would make you feel, you probably wouldn't want to.)

You'll gain freedom. Most diets deprive you of something—whether it's carbs, fat, or fun. (Can I have a blue-cheese bacon burger, hold the bun? No thanks.) In this plan, you will not feel deprived. You'll stay full. You'll eat crunchy food. You'll eat sweet food. You'll eat protein, carbs, and fat. In fact, there's even one meal during the week when you can eat anything you want. Anything. During the bulk of the week, you'll focus on foods that will charge your metabolism and control your temptations, but you'll also have the freedom and flexibility to stray just enough to keep you satisfied without ruining all the work you've already put in.

You'll gain time. On some diets, it seems like it would take less time to raise a farm of chickens and wait for the eggs to drop than it would take to plan and cook the recipes they tout. On this diet, all of the meals and recipes are low maintenance. For planning purposes, all I want you to do is take this program 2 days at a time. Because mindless noshing is the nation's number one diet buster, your best defense is to plot out a simple strategy for how and what you're going to eat each day. Every night, take 5 minutes to sketch out what and when you'll eat the next day, and you'll have deflated temptation and gained control. After reading the principles, you'll see that the New Abs Diet establishes a new paradigm for weight control. Simply:

MORE FOOD + MORE MUSCLE = LESS FLAB

Chapter 3

BURN FAT DAY AND NIGHT

How Metabolism Shapes Your Body—
And How You Can Change Yours

I N CHAPTER 2, I DISCUSSED

how most popular diets are designed to offer only short-term weight loss, and how following these programs sets you up not only to regain the weight you initially shed but to actually gain even more fat in the long run. Most diets, in fact, are not long-term fat-loss plans but long-term muscle-loss plans. The New Abs Diet is different: It's a program that helps you rev up your body's natural fat burners and keep them revved up for life.

As harmful as most diet crazes may be, diets alone aren't to blame for the obesity epidemic in America. In fact, there's plenty of blame to go around: fast food, funnel cakes, stress, sedentary lifestyles, supersizing, all-you-can-eat buffets, the demise of physical education classes, free refills, couches, movie theater popcorn, you name it. We're a society of overeaters who often hold desk jobs and would lobby to make the Bloomin' Onion its own food group. But in the battle of weight control, these are the easy targets. Instead, I'd argue, one of the reasons we keep getting fatter is that we put our faith in two things that are supposed to help us lose weight. These weight loss "double agents" reap praise for their contributions to good health, but they've also done their part in skewing the way we think about weight loss. The two culprits I blame for our obesity epidemic? Nutritional labels and exercise machines.

The Case against Calorie Counting

BEFORE YOU BUST a button, hear me out. Labels and machines both have their appropriate uses (the former for the simple knowledge of the vitamins, minerals, and ingredients in your food; the latter for getting people off their duffs and exercising). My beef with labels and machines is not what they do per se but the myth they perpetuate. Through their functions, they feed into a way of thinking about weight loss that actually makes it harder to control weight. They've turned us into a community of heavies who worship at the altar of one seemingly omnipotent number: the calorie.

With every food you eat and with every workout you finish, you look at how many calories come in and how many calories go out. It's the turnstile theory of weight loss: If you exercise away more than you take in, then you'll lose weight. Experts tell us that a pound of fat contains roughly 3,500 calories, so if you simply delete 500 calories from your daily meals, increase your daily exercise by 500 calories, or some combination thereof, you'll lose a pound of fat a week. That sounds great in theory, but in real life, the whole concept of calorie management is more likely to make you lose heart than lose weight. You hump it on the stairclimber for 30 minutes and sweat like a guest on *The O'Reilly Factor*. When you see the final readout—"Workout Completed; 300 Calories Burned!"—you feel like you've just chipped away at your belly and gotten closer to your goal. That is, until you reach for a midnight snack and see that a serving and a half of Raisin Bran also equals 300 calories. What took 30 minutes to burn takes 30 seconds to dust off during Letterman. It's a psychological diet killer.

Of course, there's nothing wrong with using nutritional labels to track what you eat or as a deterrent to stay away from high-calorie foods in the first place. And it can be helpful to use machine readouts to gauge the intensity of your exercise. But you will derail your weight loss efforts if you keep focusing on the number of calories you take in during meals and the number of calories you burn off during exercise. You need to focus, rather, on what is happening inside your body during the rest of your day—when you're working, sleeping, making love, or just sitting still right now reading this book. Right this very instant, your body is either gaining fat or losing fat. The Abs Diet will train your body to lose fat while you're sitting still, because the Abs Diet focuses on something other diet plans miss: your metabolism.

What Is "Metabolism"?

METABOLISM IS THE rate at which your body burns its way through calories just to keep itself alive—to keep your heart beating, your lungs breathing, your blood pumping, and your mind fantasizing about the Caribbean while crunching accounting figures. Your body is burning calories all the time, even while you're reading this sentence. The average woman burns about 10 calories per pound of body weight ever day; the average man, 11 per pound.

There are three main types of calorie burn that happen throughout your day. Understand how they work, and you'll understand exactly why the Abs Diet is going to turn your body into a fat-burning machine.

Calorie burn #1: The thermic effect of eating. Between 10 and 30 percent of the calories you burn each day get burned by the simple act of digesting your food. Now that's pretty cool—satisfying your food cravings actually makes you burn away calories. But not all foods are created equal: Your body uses more calories to digest protein (about 25 calories burned for every 100 calories consumed) than it does to digest fats and carbohydrates (10 to 15 calories burned for every 100 calories consumed). That's why the New Abs Diet concentrates on lean, healthy proteins. Eat more of them, in a sensible way, and you'll burn more calories.

Calorie burn #2: Exercise and movement. Another 10 to 15 percent of your calorie burn comes from moving your muscles, whether you're pressing weights overhead, running to catch the bus, or just twiddling your thumbs. Simply turning the pages of this book will burn calories.

Calorie burn #3: Basal metabolism. This one's the biggie. Your basal, or resting, metabolism refers to the calories you're burning when you're doing nothing at all. Sleeping, watching TV, sitting through yet another mind-numbing presentation on corporate profit-and-loss statements—you're burning calories all the while. In fact, between 60 and 80 percent of your daily calories

(continued on page 42)

What the Heck Is . . . High Cholesterol?

Cholesterol is a soft, waxy substance found among the lipids (fats) in the bloodstream and in all your body's cells. For all the bad press it gets, the fact is that you need cholesterol, because your body uses it to form cell membranes, create hormones, and perform several other crucial maintenance operations. But a high level of cholesterol in the blood—hypercholesterolemia—is a major risk factor for coronary heart disease, which leads to heart attack.

You get cholesterol in two ways. The body—mainly the liver—produces varying amounts, usually about 1,000 milligrams a day. But when you consume foods high in saturated fats—particularly trans fats—your body goes cholesterol crazy, pumping out more than you could ever use. (Some foods also contain cholesterol, especially egg yolks, meat, poultry, fish, seafood, and whole-milk dairy products. But the majority of it, and the stuff I want you to focus on, is made by your own body.)

Some of the excess cholesterol in your bloodstream is removed from the body through the liver. But some of it winds up exactly where you don't want it—along the walls of your arteries, where it combines with other substances to form plaque. Plaque is wack for several reasons: First, it raises blood pressure by making your heart work harder to get blood through your suddenly narrower vessels, which can eventually wear out your ticker. Second, plaque can break off its little perch and tumble through your bloodstream, eventually forming a clot that can lead to stroke, paralysis, death, and other annoyances.

Inside your body, a war is raging right now between two factions of specialized sherpas called lipoproteins that are moving cholesterol around your insides according to their own specialized agendas. There are several kinds, but the ones to focus on are the Jekyll and Hyde of health, HDL (high-density or "helpful" lipoprotein) and LDL (low-density or "lazy" lipoprotein) cholesterol.

The good guy: HDL cholesterol. About one-fourth to one-third of blood cholesterol is carried by helpful HDL. HDL wants to help you out by picking up cholesterol and getting it the hell out of your bloodstream by carrying it back to the liver, where it's passed from the body. That's good. Some experts believe that HDL removes excess cholesterol from plaques and thus slows their growth. That's really good. A high HDL level—above 60 milligrams per deciliter (mg/dL)—seems to protect against heart attack. The opposite is also true: A low HDL level—less than 40 milligrams per deciliter (mg/dL)—indicates a greater risk. A low HDL cholesterol level may also raise stroke risk.

The bad guy: LDL cholesterol. Lazy LDL has no interest at all in helping you out. LDL just wants to stick cholesterol in the most convenient place it can find, meaning your arteries. LDL doesn't care that too much cholesterol lining your arteries causes a buildup of plaque, a condition known as atherosclerosis. A high level of LDL cholesterol (160 mg/dL and above) reflects an increased risk of heart disease. Lower levels of LDL cholesterol reflect a lower risk of heart disease.

The other bad guy: Triglycerides. These are a kind of fat in your blood that your body uses for energy. You need it, but when you have too much, you increase your risk for abdominal fat, diabetes, high bloosd pressure, even low HDL. A triglyceride check should be part of your regular cholesterol blood work. Ask for it if it isn't. A good triglyceride level is below 150 mg/dl. Triglycerides rise when you eat more calories than you burn off, drink a lot of alcohol or consume trans fats typically found in baked goods and chips.

Simply put, HDL is trying to come to your aid, while LDL and excess triglycerides are just sitting there, laughing at you. So whose side are you on? If you want to lower your triglycerides and boost HDL, start stocking up on the Abs Diet Powerfoods and follow the guidelines of the Abs Diet Workout. Here are some more quick ideas on beating the bad guys for good:

Drop 10 pounds. For every pound of fat you lose, your good HDL rises 1 percent.

Butt out. Tobacco smoking is one of the six major risk factors of heart disease that you can change or treat. Smoking lowers HDL cholesterol levels. If your partner smokes, you're in danger, too. A recent study at Florida State University found that exposing nonsmokers to tobacco smoke in a typical tavern depressed their HDL levels up to 20 percent for up to two days.

Drink up or quit. In some studies, moderate use of alcohol is linked with higher HDL cholesterol levels. But take it easy there, Dino. People who consume moderate amounts of alcohol (an average of one drink per day for women and one or two drinks a day for men) have a lower risk of heart disease, but increased consumption of alcohol can bring other health dangers, such as alcoholism, high blood pressure, obesity, and cancer. And alcohol raises triglyceride levels. If you have high tris, cutting out drinking is a sure way to bring them down.

Johnny B good. A B vitamin called niacin reduces LDL cholesterol at the same time it raises beneficial HDL. In fact, niacin can be more effective at treating these things than popular cholesterol-busting drugs, which tend to act more generally on total cholesterol and gross LDL. (Be careful, though. While the niacin you get

(continued)

ABS DIET HEALTH BULLETIN

What the Heck Is . . . High Cholesterol? (cont.)

from foods and over-the-counter vitamins is fine, super-high doses of niacin can have serious side effects and should be taken only under a doctor's supervision.)

Tea it up. Three recent studies confirm that drinking green tea can help lower your cholesterol level and reduce your risk of developing cancer. In a 12-week trial of 240 men and women, researchers at Vanderbilt University found that drinking the equivalent of 7 cups of green tea a day can help lower LDL cholesterol levels by 16 percent. Seven cups a day is a lot of tea, but even 1 or 2 cups a day could have a beneficial impact. Meanwhile, researchers at the University of Rochester recently determined that green tea extract can help prevent the growth of cancer cells, and Medical College of Ohio researchers found that a compound called EGCG in green tea may help slow or stop the progression of bladder cancer.

Go for the grapefruit. If you want to make one simple dietary change for better health, the best thing you can do is eat a single white or ruby grapefruit every day. Grapefruit is gaining ground as a powerful food. New research shows that it can fight heart disease and cancer, trigger your body to lose weight, and even help you get a better night's sleep. A grapefruit a day can lower your total cholesterol and LDL cholesterol levels by 8 and 11 percent, respectively.

Take a hike. Studies at Auburn University and the Cooper Institute in Dallas show that regular moderate exercise boosts HDL levels and reduces artery inflammation.

Cram in the cranberry. Researchers at the University of Scranton in Pennsylvania found that men who drank three glasses of cranberry juice daily raised their HDL cholesterol levels by 10 percent, which in turn lowered their risk of heart disease by 40 percent. Plant compounds called polyphenols are believed to be responsible for the effect. (Note: Cranberry juice often comes diluted, so make sure the label says that it contains at least 27 percent cranberry juice.)

Spread some on. Instead of butter or margarine, try Benecol spread. It contains stanol ester, a plant substance that inhibits cholesterol absorption. A study at the Mayo Clinic found that people eating 4½ tablespoons of Benecol daily lowered their LDL cholesterol by 14 percent in 8 weeks. When they stopped using it, their LDL returned to previous levels. Benecol can also be used for cooking.

Gain with grains and beans. Researchers at St. Michael's Hospital in Toronto had people add several servings of foods like whole grains, nuts, and beans to their diets each day. One month later, the test subjects' LDL cholesterol levels were nearly 30 percent lower than when the trial began. In another study, this one at Tulane University, researchers found that people who ate four or more servings a week had a 22 percent lower risk of developing heart disease (and 75 percent fewer camping companions) than less-than-once-a-week bean eaters.

Don't let your tank hit empty. A study in the *British Medical Journal* found that people who eat six or more small meals a day have 5 percent lower cholesterol levels than those who eat one or two large meals. That's enough to shrink your risk of heart disease by 10 to 20 percent.

Refrain from fries. In a study published in the *New England Journal of Medicine,* the exercise and nutritional habits of 80,000 women were recorded for 14 years. The researchers found that the most important correlate of heart disease was the women's dietary intake of foods containing trans fatty acids, mutated forms of fat that lower HDL and increase LDL. Some of the worst offenders are french fries.

Sow your oats. In a University of Connecticut study, men with high cholesterol who ate oat bran cookies daily for 8 weeks dropped their levels of LDL cholesterol by more than 20 percent. So eat more oat bran fiber, such as oatmeal or Cheerios. A study in the *American Journal of Clinical Nutrition* reports that two servings of whole-grain cereal (Cheerios count) a day can reduce a man's risk of dying of heart disease by nearly 20 percent.

Fortify with folic acid. A study published in the *British Medical Journal* found that people who consume the recommended amount of folic acid each day have a 16 percent lower risk of heart disease than those whose diets are lacking in this B vitamin. Good sources of folic acid include asparagus, broccoli, and fortified cereal.

Order a chef's salad. Leafy greens and egg yolks are both good sources of lutein, a phytochemical that carries heart disease–fighting antioxidants to your cells and tissues.

Be a sponge. Loma Linda University researchers found that drinking five or more 8-ounce glasses of water a day could help lower your risk of heart disease by up to 60 percent—exactly the same drop you get from stopping smoking, lowering your LDL cholesterol numbers, exercising, or losing a little weight.

Give yourself bad breath. In addition to lowering cholesterol and helping to fight off infection, eating garlic may help limit damage to your heart after a heart attack or heart surgery. Researchers in India found that animals that were fed garlic regularly had more heart-protecting antioxidants in their blood than animals that weren't.

Crank up the chromium. According to new research from Harvard, men with low levels of chromium in their systems are significantly more likely to develop heart problems. You need between 200 and 400 micrograms of chromium per day—more than you're likely to get from your regular diet. Look for a supplement labeled chromium picolinate; it's the most easily absorbed by the body.

Snack on nuts. Harvard researchers found that men who replaced 127 calories of carbohydrates—that's about 14 Baked Lay's potato chips—with 1 ounce of nuts decreased their risk of heart disease by 30 percent.

are burned up just doing nothing. That's because your body is constantly in motion: Your heart is beating, your lungs are breathing, and your cells are dividing, all the time, even when you sleep.

Add up the percentages and you'll see that the majority of your daily calorie burn comes from physiological functions that you don't even think about—the thermic effect of eating and your basal metabolism. While exercise is important, you need to realize that the calories you burn off during exercise aren't important. Let me repeat that: Exercise is important, but the calories you burn off during exercise aren't important. That's why the exercise program we outline in the New Abs Diet is designed to alter your basal metabolism, turning your downtime into fat-burning time. And it's why the food choices

---

ABS DIET SUCCESS STORY

"The Proof Is in the Pants!"

Name: Jessica Guff

Age: 43

Height: 5'4"

Starting weight: 130

Six weeks later: 120

Jessica Guff doesn't believe in stepping on a scale. See, numbers don't give a total health picture, Guff says. What really matters is how you view yourself—not to mention how others view you, too. Take the time she was walking into a client's office. The people there hadn't seen her for a couple of weeks, and one employee said to another, "Who's that skinny woman over there?"

"It's Jessica," the other employee told her. "She's on this thing called the Abs Diet."

That exchange took place just 2 weeks after Guff started the Abs Diet—and she felt the effects immediately. Guff, 43, who runs marathons, has always been in good shape. But the effect of having two kids had taken a toll on her belly. "I was in pretty good shape, except for my stomach," she says. "But since going on the plan, I really noticed a difference. I could probably crunch walnuts with my abs."

The key for Guff was changing the way she approached eating. Sacrificing her own eating habits to get her kids out the door and keep up with her fitness training, she'd start the day with tea—and often little else. "I used to go out and run without eating anything, and that was really stupid," Guff says. "I was horrified to learn the truth—that

we outline for you are designed to maximize the number of calories you burn simply by eating and digesting. I want you to forget about the calories you're burning during those 30 minutes in the gym and concentrate on the calories you're burning the other 23½ hours a day.

In effect, the New Abs Diet is going to change your body into a fat-frying dynamo by several means.

Changing the Way You Exercise

HAVE YOU EVER seen a gym at rush hour? Everyone hovers around the treadmills, elliptical trainers, and stationary bikes. Signs warn you of 20-minute

exercising on an empty stomach causes you to burn muscle, not fat." But the simple strategies of the Abs Diet changed all that. "Now I'm having smoothies for breakfast, and it's made me fitter and stoked up my energy," Guff says.

Guff says she couldn't do a program in which she'd have to count calories or weigh food. "What I love about the Abs Diet is the flexibility," she says. "All I have to remember is the catchy acronym—ABS DIET POWER—and I can remember the 12 powerfoods."

The results: She's leaner—and stronger. When her 56-pound daughter fell asleep on the couch, Guff was the one who picked her up and carried her to bed. "I thought, either I'm getting stronger or she's losing weight," she says.

And she's also more confident. "When women look at other women, they look at their boobs, their butts, and their waists—especially women who've had children. Every woman who's had a child cares about having a flat stomach."

But the true measure of her success came in the form of a pair of green satin cargo pants. Guff says, "They're kinda hot, but my stomach shows when I wear them. I have two kids, so I have no business flashing my midsection." But after 2 weeks on the plan, she decided to put them to the public test.

"All these people started complimenting me. A guy I went to college with said, 'Nice outfit.' My husband said I looked great," Guff says. "I'm going out tonight and I'm wearing the pants again."

maximums so that the next sweat seeker can have his turn. It seems like everyone wants a cardiovascular, aerobic workout. The more you sweat, the more calories you burn, the more weight you lose, right? In a way, yes, the headphone-and-Lycra set is right. Cardiovascular exercise—steady-state endurance exercises, like running, biking, and swimming—burns a lot of calories. In fact, it often burns more than other forms of exercise like strength training or trendier workouts like yoga or Pilates. But when it comes to weight control, aerobic exercise is more overrated than the fall TV lineup. Why? For one reason: Aerobic exercise builds little (if any) muscle—and muscle is the key component of a speedy metabolism. Muscle eats fat; again, add 1 pound of muscle, and your body burns up to an additional 50 calories a day just to keep that muscle alive. Add 6 pounds of muscle, and suddenly you're burning up to 300 more calories each day just by sitting still.

Here's the problem with low-intensity aerobic exercise. Just like a car can't run without gas or a kite can't fly without wind, a body can't function without food. It's the fuel that helps you run, lift, and have the legs to make love all night long. Generally, during exercise, your body calls upon glycogen (the stored form of carbohydrate in muscles and the liver), fat, and in some cases protein. When you're doing low-intensity aerobic exercise like jogging, your body primarily uses fat and glycogen (carbohydrates) for fuel. When it continues at longer periods (20 minutes or more), your body drifts into depletion: You exhaust your first-tier energy sources (your glycogen stores), and your body hunts around for the easiest source of energy it can find—protein. Your body actually begins to eat up muscle tissue, converting the protein stored in your muscles into energy you need to keep going. Once your body reaches that plateau, it burns up 5 to 6 grams of protein for every 30 minutes of ongoing exercise. (That's roughly the amount of protein you'll find in a hard-boiled egg.) By burning protein, you're not only missing an opportunity to burn fat but also losing all-important and powerful muscle. So aerobic exercise actually decreases muscle mass. Decreased muscle mass ultimately slows down your metabolism, making it easier for you to gain weight.

Now here's a shocking fact: When early studies compared cardio exercise to weight training, researchers learned that people who did aerobics burned more calories during exercise than those who lifted weights. You'd assume, then, that aerobic exercise was the way to go. But that's not the end of the story.

It turns out that while lifters didn't burn as many calories during their workouts as the folks who ran or biked, they burned far more calories over the course of the next several hours. This phenomenon is known as the afterburn—the additional calories your body burns off in the hours and days after a workout. When researchers looked at the metabolic increases after exercise, they found that the increased metabolic effect of aerobics lasted only 30 to 60 minutes. The effects of weight training lasted as long as 48 hours. That's 48 hours during which the body was burning additional fat. Over the long term, both groups lost weight, but those who practiced strength training lost only fat, while the runners and bikers lost muscle mass as well. The message: Aerobic exercise essentially burns only at the time of the workout. Strength training burns calories long after you leave the gym, while you sleep, and maybe all the way until your next workout. Plus, the extra muscle you build through strength training means that in the long term your body keeps burning calories at rest just to keep that new muscle alive.

That raises a question. What aspect of strength training creates the long afterburn? Most likely, it's the process of muscle repair. Weight lifting causes your muscle tissues to break down and rebuild themselves at a higher rate than normal. (Muscles are always breaking down and rebuilding; strength training simply accelerates the process.) That breakdown and rebuilding takes a lot of energy and could be what accounts for the long period of calorie burning. In fact, a Finnish study found that protein synthesis (the process that builds bigger muscles) increases 21 percent 3 hours after a workout.

The good news is that you don't have to lift like a linebacker to see the results. A recent Ohio University study found that a short but hard workout had the same effect as longer workouts. Using a circuit of three exercises in a row for 31 minutes, the subjects were still burning more calories than normal 38 hours after the workout. (The New Abs Diet Workout is designed along similar principles, to mimic these results.) Even very brief strength workouts are worth your effort on days when you don't have a lot of time. Researchers at the University of Southern Maine calculated that performing just one 8-minute-long circuit of eight exercises burns up to 231 calories, on par with the number you would burn by running a 6-minute mile pace for the same duration.

As I said earlier, building muscle increases your metabolism so much that you burn up to 50 calories per day per pound of muscle you have. The more muscle you have, the easier it is for you to lose fat. That's why one of the components of the plan includes an exercise program that will help you add the muscle you need to burn fat and reshape your body. And it also points to one of the reasons why you should de-emphasize cardiovascular, aerobic exercise if you want to lose fat: because it depletes your body's store of fat-burning muscle.

Now, before you start thinking I'm some sort of anti-aerobics fanatic, let me clarify a few things: I run almost daily, and I've even completed the New York City Marathon. Aerobic exercise burns calories, it helps control stress, and it improves your cardiovascular fitness. It also helps lower blood pressure and improve your cholesterol profile. If your choice is aerobic exercise or no exercise, for Pete's sake get out there and run. But when it comes to long-term weight management, I'll take gym iron over road rubber any day.

Changing the Way You Eat

FEW THINGS IN American society have failed more often than diets. I think there's an explanation for the high failure rate. For one, many diets have revolved around low-fat menus. I'll discuss fat in a later chapter, but one of the problems with low-fat diets is that they can suppress the manufacture of testosterone, the hormone that contributes to the growth of muscle and the burning of fat. When testosterone levels are low, your body stores fat like squirrels store nuts. In one study, men with higher testosterone were 75 percent less likely to be obese than men with lower levels of testosterone. Many diets also fail because they don't take advantage of the single most powerful nutrient for building muscle and increasing your metabolism: protein.

Protein—in proportion with foods from other groups—works in two primary ways. First, eating more protein cranks up the thermic effect of digestion by as much as one-third. Second, protein is also the nutrient that builds calorie-consuming muscle. In effect, you get a double burn—while you're digesting food and later, as it helps build muscle. In the New Abs Diet, you'll emphasize protein for these very reasons, but you'll also emphasize the most powerful sources of protein. A Danish study published in the *American Journal of Clinical Nutrition* put a group of men on diets that were high in protein either from pork or from soy. They found that men on the animal protein diet burned 2 percent more calories during a 24-hour period than men on the soy protein diet.

That's 50 calories a day if you're eating a 2,500-calorie diet. In other words, if you want to burn calories, tenderloin is better than tofu.

Changing the Way You Think About the Word "Diet"

HERE'S A TYPICAL diet scenario: You nibble on a piece of toast for breakfast and baby carrots for lunch, and you figure that puts you well ahead of the calorie-counting game. By dinner, though, you've got so many onion rings jammed into your mouth that you look like Dizzy Gillespie. If you're so restricted in what you can eat, you'll eventually act like a rebellious teen and break the rules. While most diets say "no" more than your boss at review time, the New Abs Diet says "yes." Most diets are about restricting. This one is about fueling.

For years—or maybe for all your life—you've probably had one notion about what dieting needs to be. Restrict your foods, eat like a supermodel, sweat on the treadmill, and you'll lose fat. In reality, those could be the very reasons why you couldn't lose weight. It's why you gained back what you lost. It's the reason why your speedboat metabolism may have geared down to that of an anchored barge. It's why you don't see much progress when you try new weight loss programs. And it's why the only real recipe many diet plans offer is a recipe for pecan-encrusted failure. What the New Abs Diet will do is reprogram your circuitry. You'll stop thinking about every calorie and start thinking about how best to burn calories. Once you master that, your body will be equipped with all the tools it needs to strip away fat—and show off your abs.

Chapter 4

HOW THE NEW ABS DIET WORKS
What Your Last Meal Is Doing to Your Body Right Now

IN THE CRUDEST FORM, THE way in which food travels through your body seems simple. There's one way in and one way out, and anything left behind snowballs into a mound of fat on your gut, over your hips, or under your chin. In reality, the travel patterns of your breakfast, lunch, and dinner flow more like a Los Angeles interstate system than anything else. You've got the traffic jams (clogged arteries) and the occasional drive-by shootings (indigestion), but you also have a complex network of roads that shuttle nutrients to and from vital organs and tissues. Your ability to lose weight and gain muscle largely depends on how and when you fuel your body to work in that system.

In the previous chapter, I showed how the key to effective weight management was concentrating on your body's calorie burn—not on how effectively you burn calories while exercising but on how effectively you burn calories when you're not exercising. Additionally, I explained a little about how the foods you eat can affect your body's daily calorie burn. Before I explain the how-tos of the New Abs Diet, you should know the most important substances and nutrients that affect the way your body processes food.

Protein: The MVP

IN SPORTS, FEW things are as valued as versatility—a center who can rebound and shoot, a quarterback who runs as well as he passes, a shortstop who can belt homers and flash leather. In your body, protein is the most versatile player on your nutrient team. It comes in many forms and does so many things well—all without a $254 million contract.

▶ Protein builds the framework of your body, including muscles, organs, bones, and connective tissues.

▶ In the form of enzymes, it helps your body digest food.

▶ As a hormone, it tells your body when to use food as energy and when to store it as fat.

▶ It transports oxygen through your blood to your muscles and organs.

ABS DIET SUCCESS STORY

"The Abs Diet Helped Me Cheat Death!"

Name: Dan Shea

Age: 40

Height: 5'7"

Starting weight: 226

Six weeks later: 207

Dan Shea had seen what happens to a man who doesn't take charge of his weight and his health, and he didn't want it to happen to him. His own dad—a once-fit airborne ranger who used to be in incredible shape—was now, at age 70, on the verge of losing a foot to diabetes. Shea wanted to plot a different course: "I want to be skiing when I'm 70," he says.

But at 40 years old, 5 feet 7 inches, and 226 pounds, Shea knew he had to make a change—a 60-pound change. He had a 13-year-old daughter he wanted to watch grow up, and at the rate he was going, he was a heart attack waiting to happen. So he started the Abs Diet and immediately took to it. He realized the importance of eating

▶ As an antibody, it protects you from illness when viruses and bacteria launch an attack.

So protein is critical for helping your body to function at optimum levels. But we've made protein the foundation of the New Abs Diet for four other very important reasons.

1. It tastes good. Juicy steaks. Sliced smoked turkey. Roasted pork loin. Steamed lobster. Peanut butter. The New Abs Diet is built around the foods you crave, so it's a program you're not going to have to stick to; it's a program you're going to want to stick to.

2. It burns calories even as you're indulging in it. Food contains energy in the form of chemical bonds, but your body can't use them in that form. Your body has to break down the food and extract energy from that chemical bond; that process of extracting energy itself

---

often—making sure he had a mid-morning snack consisting of some powerfoods. "Even though I wasn't hungry, I ate it," he says. "It was like fighting years of dietary knowledge to have that snack. I wasn't hungry yet, but if I hadn't eaten, I'd have been starving at lunch."

But his biggest affection is for the Abs Diet smoothies that he makes with low-fat yogurt, low-fat milk, some fruit, and a scoop of protein powder. "Best damn thing on the planet, like going to Dairy Queen," Shea says. "For fun, I'd layer it with a couple of tablespoons of fat-free, sugar-free whipped topping. My life is all about smoothies now. If I could have a blender in my office, I'd have them three times a day."

Shea lost 19 pounds on the plan and now has made the Abs Diet his regular eating and nutritional plan. "I look great, or so my wife tells me. My pants are much looser, and I need a new belt. I tuck in my shirts now. I walk taller somehow, stand taller. My confidence level has been boosted. In fact, I had an interview for a position for which I was way underqualified, yet I was short-listed and came quite close to getting it, based largely on my strength of presence," Shea says. "I've lost in my gut and butt, but mainly my man breasts are now less Dolly Parton and more Gwyneth Paltrow. I know this is a great plan, and I know I'm going to reach my goal. I mean, I'm in it for the long haul, and this is a plan that is easy to do for the long term."

requires energy, so your body's burning more calories to do it. That's the thermic effect of eating, as I explained in Chapter 3, and protein pushes the thermic effect into high gear. It takes almost two times more energy to break down protein than it does to break down carbohydrates. So when you feed your body a greater amount of protein, your body automatically burns more calories throughout the day. When Arizona State University researchers compared the benefits of a high-protein diet with those of a high-carbohydrate diet, they found that people who ate a high-protein diet burned more than twice as many calories in the hours after their meals as those eating predominantly carbs.

3. It keeps you feeling satisfied. Research has shown that if you base your meals around protein, you'll feel fuller faster. Consider one study in the *European Journal of Clinical Nutrition*. Subjects downed one type of four different kinds of shakes—60 percent protein, 60 percent carbohydrate, 60 percent fat, or a mixture with equal amounts of all three. Then they were offered lunch. The subjects who had either the high-protein or mixed-nutrient shakes ate the least for lunch. The shakes they had downed contained the same number of calories, but the protein made them feel fuller and eat less at lunchtime.

4. It builds muscle and keeps your body burning fat all day. Remember, more muscle burns more fat. When you lift and lower weights, you create microscopic tears in your muscles. To repair the tears, protein acts like the Red Cross in a federal disaster area. Your body parachutes in new protein to assess the damage and repair the muscle. Proteins fortify the original cell structure by building new muscle fibers.

This whole process through which proteins make new muscle fibers after a workout can last anywhere from 24 to 48 hours. So if you lift weights 3 days a week—triggering proteins to rush in and repair your muscles—your body essentially stays in muscle-building, and thus fat-burning, mode every day.

As you know, protein comes in many forms—such as turkey, beef, fish, nuts, and tofu. You want to concentrate on the proteins that best help build your muscles. Research has shown that animal protein builds muscle better than soy or vegetable protein does. So poultry, fish, and lean cuts of beef or pork are a better choice than tofu or other soy-based products. If you're the kind of guy who likes to count, you'll want to shoot for about 1 gram of protein per pound of body weight per day—that's roughly the amount of protein your body can use every day. For a 160-pound man, that's 160 grams (g) of protein a day, which would break down into something like this:

3   eggs (18 g)

2   cups of 1 percent milk (16 g)

1   cup of cottage cheese (28 g)

1   roast beef sandwich (28 g)

2½ ounces of peanuts (16 g)

8   ounces of chicken breast (54 g)

Combine those four reasons—an easy and delicious eating plan, more calorie burn, less calorie intake, and more fat-burning muscle—and you can easily see how a high-protein diet translates into weight loss. In a Danish study, researchers put 65 subjects on a 12 percent protein diet, a 25 percent protein diet, or no diet (the control group). In the first two groups, the same percentage of calories—about 30 percent—came from fat. While the low-protein dieters lost an average of more than 11 pounds, the high-protein subjects lost an average of 20 pounds and ate fewer calories than the low-protein group.

The more amazing statistic wasn't how much they lost but where they lost it: The high-protein dieters also lost twice as much abdominal fat. One reason may be that a high-protein diet helps your body control its levels of cortisol, a stress hormone that causes fat to converge in the abdominal region.

Fat: Underrated, Understand?

WHEN YOU THINK of fat, you probably think of foods that have a lot of fat—or people who do. After a few years with some extra pounds, the only thing you know about fat is that you're tired of it and want to get rid of it forever. But it's probably one of your body's most misunderstood dietary nutrients, stemming from a widely held but misguided belief that fat should take much of the blame for our obesity epidemic.

(continued on page 58)

What the Heck Is . . . Diabetes?

Diabetes is a devastating disease that is reaching epidemic proportions. Twenty-four million Americans are living with diabetes and up to 54 million may have prediabetes, the precursor to type 2 diabetes. Diabetes is the seventh leading cause of death in the US, but because it often goes undiagnosed, it is probably responsible for many more deaths. It's a leading cause of heart disease, kidney disease, and stroke, and its other complications include blindness, amputation, sexual dysfunction, and nerve damage. And the incidence of type 2—the kind of diabetes that people develop over time versus type 1 or juvenile diabetes—has grown 32 percent faster among American men than among American women in the past quarter-century. According to the Centers for Disease Control, someone with diabetes is twice as likely to die as someone the same age without diabetes. Fortunately, type 2 diabetes is also highly preventable (even reversible) and the New Abs Diet and the New Abs Diet Workout are near-perfect prescriptions.

Diabetes works like this: Your digestive system turns brunch into glucose—the form of sugar your body uses for energy—and sends it into the bloodstream. When the glucose hits, your pancreas—a large gland located near your stomach—produces insulin, a hormone, and sends that into the bloodstream as well. Insulin is your body's air traffic controller: It takes command of all your glucose and directs it into your cells, where it can be used for rebuilding muscle, for keeping your heart pumping and your brain thinking, or for doing the macarena (if you're the type to do the macarena, that is).

But over time, bad health habits can take a toll on your flight command center. Overeating, particularly eating high-glycemic index foods, floods your body with massive amounts of glucose time and time again. Like any air traffic controller, insulin can become overwhelmed when it's asked to do too much all at one time, and eventually it burns out. Insulin loses its ability to tell cells how to properly utilize the glucose in your blood—a condition known as insulin resistance. After several years, the pancreas gets fed up with producing all that ineffective insulin and begins to produce less than you need. This is called type 2, or adult-onset, diabetes. (Type 1 is caused by a defect in the pancreas.) Given that poor diet is the major risk factor for type 2 diabetes, it's no surprise that 80 percent of people with the disease are overweight. Glucose builds up in the blood, overflows into the urine, and passes out of the body. Thus, the body loses its main source of fuel even though the blood contains large amounts of glucose.

Two bad things happen: First, you start to lose energy, and your body starts to have trouble maintaining itself. You feel fatigue and unusual thirst, and you begin losing weight for no apparent reason; you get sick more often, and injuries are slow to heal, because your body is losing its ability to maintain itself. Second, the sugar that is hanging around in your blood begins to damage the tiny blood vessels and nerves throughout your body, particularly in your extremities and vital organs. Blindness, impotence, numbness, and heart damage ensue.

But type 2 diabetes is a highly preventable disease. Exercising and eating right are the two best ways to manage it—and what a coincidence, that's just what this book is intended to teach you to do. So adopt the principles of the New Abs Diet and the New Abs Diet Workout, and while you're at it, consider these additional steps:

Get mushy. Oatmeal is high in soluble fiber, which may decrease your risk of heart disease, some cancers, diverticulitis, and diabetes. Mix it up: Eat oatmeal with berries and nuts one day, and have eggs and meat another.

Climb. Yale researchers found that men with insulin resistance—a risk factor for diabetes and heart disease—who exercised on a stairclimber for 45 minutes 4 days a week improved their sensitivity to insulin by 43 percent in 6 weeks.

Cruise the Mediterranean. Eating a Mediterranean-style diet—that is, whole grains, fresh vegetables, and oily fish—maximizes your metabolism and slashes diabetes risk. A 2008 study of 13,380 people reported in the *British Medical Journal* showed that those who adhered closely to a Mediterranean diet had a 35 percent lower risk of diabetes than those who did not consistently follow such an eating style.

Steal from the teacher. Researchers at the National Public Health Institute in Helsinki, Finland, studied the diets of 60,000 men and women over the course of a year and found that individuals who ate apples the most frequently were 12 percent less likely to die during the course of the study than those who rarely bit into a McIntosh or Granny Smith. In particular, they cut their risk of diabetes by 27 percent.

Eat more E. In the alphabet soup of vitamins, E is the one that may prevent the big D. When Finnish researchers evaluated the diets of 944 men, they found that those with the highest vitamin E intake had a 22 percent lower risk of diabetes than men with the lowest intake. Vitamin E may also prevent the free-radical damage that plays a role in the complications caused by diabetes.

In the 1980s, the US government released nutritional guidelines that essentially said we should base our diets on potatoes, rice, cereal, and pasta and minimize the foods with a lot of fat and protein. That gave way to the idea that fat makes you fat. And that gave way to a new breed of diets that said if you limit the fat in what you eat, you'll limit the fat that exercises squatter's rights on your gut. But that line of thinking didn't hold out when researchers tried to find links between low-fat diets and obesity. In 1998, for example, two prominent obesity researchers estimated that if you took only 10 percent of your calories from fat, you'd lose 16 grams of fat a day—a loss of 50 pounds in a year. But when a Harvard epidemiologist, Walter Willett, tried to find evidence that this occurred, he couldn't find any link between people who lost weight and the fact that they were on a low-fat diet. In fact, in some studies lasting a year or more, groups of people showed weight gains on low-fat diets. Willett speculated that there was a mechanism responsible for this: When the body is on a low-fat diet for a long period, it stops losing weight.

Part of the reason our bodies rebel against low-fat diets is that we need fat. For instance, fat plays a vital role in the delivery of vitamins A, D, E, and K—nutrients stored in fatty tissue and the liver until your body needs them. Fat also helps produce testosterone, which helps trigger muscle growth. And fat, like protein, helps keep you satisfied and controls your appetite. In fact, if we've learned anything about weight loss over the past several years, it's that reducing your fat intake doesn't necessarily do a darn thing to decrease your body fat. One small study, for instance, compared a high-carbohydrate diet and a high-fat diet. The researchers found that the group with the high-fat diet experienced less muscle loss than the other group. The researchers theorized that muscle protein was being spared by the higher-fat diet because fatty acids, more so than carbs, were being harnessed and used for energy.

The truth is that reasonable amounts of fat can actually help you lose weight. In a study from the *International Journal of Obesity*, researchers at Boston's Brigham and Women's Hospital and Harvard Medical School put 101 overweight people on either a low-fat diet (fat was 20 percent of the total calories) or a moderate-fat diet (35 percent of calories) and followed them for 18 months. Both groups lost weight at first, but after a year and a half, the moderate-fat group had lost an average of 9 pounds per person, whereas the low-fat dieters had gained 6 pounds. The results suggest that a healthy amount of fat is a factor in keeping your weight under control.

Here's a primer on the fats in your life.

Trans fat: BAD. You won't find trans fatty acids listed on most food labels, even though there are more than 40,000 packaged foods that contain this type of fat. You won't find it listed because it's so bad for you that food manufacturers have fought for years to keep it off ingredient labels. In 2003, the US Food and Drug Administration finally adopted regulations requiring manufacturers to include trans fat content on their packaging, but the regulations will be phased in over the next few years. For now, you have to be a smart food consumer to spot where the danger lies.

Trans fats were invented by grocery manufacturers in the 1950s as a way of appealing to our natural cravings for fatty foods. But there's nothing natural about trans fats—they're cholesterol-raising, heart-weakening, diabetes-causing, belly-building chemicals that, for the most part, didn't even exist until the middle of the last century, and some studies have linked them to an estimated 30,000 premature deaths in this country every year. In one Harvard study, researchers found that getting just 3 percent of your daily calories from trans fats increased your risk of heart disease by 50 percent. Three percent of your daily calories equals about 7 grams of trans fats—that's roughly the amount in a single order of fries. Americans eat an average of between 3 and 10 grams of trans fats every day.

To understand what trans fats are, picture a bottle of vegetable oil and a stick of margarine. At room temperature, the vegetable oil is a liquid, the margarine a solid. Now, if you baked cookies using vegetable oil, they'd be pretty greasy. And who would want to buy a cookie swimming in oil? So to create cookies—and cakes, nachos, chips, pies, muffins, doughnuts, waffles, and many, many other foods we consume daily—manufacturers heat the oil to very high temperatures and infuse it with hydrogen. That hydrogen bonds with the oil to create an entirely new form of fat—trans fat—that stays solid at room temperature. Vegetable oil becomes margarine. And now foods that might normally be healthy—but maybe not as tasty—become fat bombs.

Since these trans fats don't exist in nature, your body has a hell of a time processing them. Once consumed, trans fats are free to cause all sorts of mischief inside you. They raise the number of LDL (bad) cholesterol particles in your bloodstream and lower your HDL (good) cholesterol. They also raise blood levels of other lipoproteins; the more lipoprotein you have in your bloodstream, the greater your risk of heart disease. Increased consumption of trans fats has also been linked to increased risk of diabetes and cancer.

Yet trans fats are added to a shocking number of foods. They appear on food labels as partially hydrogenated oil—usually vegetable or palm oil. Go look in your pantry and freezer right now, and you won't believe how many foods include them. Crackers. Popcorn. Cookies. Fish sticks. Cheese spreads. Candy bars. Frozen waffles. Stuffing. Even foods you might assume are healthy—like bran muffins, cereals, and nondairy creamers—are often loaded with trans fats. And because they hide in foods that look like they're low in fat, such as Wheat Thins, these fats are making you unhealthy without your even knowing it.

Take control of your trans fat intake. Check the ingredient labels on all the packaged foods you buy, and if you see partially hydrogenated oil on the label, consider finding an alternative. Even foods that seem bad for you can have healthy versions: McCain's shoestring french fries, Ruffles Natural reduced-fat chips, Wheatables reduced-fat crackers, and Dove dark chocolate bars are just a few of the "bad for you" snacks that are actually free of trans fats. And remember—the higher up on the ingredients list partially hydrogenated oil is, the worse the food is for you. You might not be able to avoid trans fats entirely, but you can choose foods with a minimal amount of the stuff.

The other way to avoid trans fats is to avoid ordering fried foods. Because trans fats spoil less easily than natural fats and are easier to ship and

How to Choose a Multivitamin

Multivitamins are good insurance for the day you don't get the daily maximum amount of nutrients. Look for one with a concentration of chromium and vitamins B6 and B12. Chromium improves your body's ability to convert amino acids into muscle. A University of Maryland study found that men who exercised regularly and took 200 micrograms of chromium a day added more muscle and lost significantly more body fat than lifters not taking the supplement. Also, because hard workouts deplete your B vitamins, it's good to find vitamins with high doses, like Solaray Men's Golden Multi-Vita-Min, which has megadoses of vitamins B6 and B12, plus your entire daily allowance of endurance-boosting zinc.

store, almost all fried commercial foods are now fried in trans fats rather than natural oils. Fish and chips, tortillas, fried chicken—all of it is packed with belly-building trans fats. Order food baked or broiled whenever possible. And avoid fast-food joints, where nearly every food option is loaded with trans fats; drive-through restaurants ought to come complete with drive-through cardiology clinics.

For more on trans fats—where they come from, how they act inside your body, and how to fight back, see the Special Report on page 119. In the meantime:

AVOID

Margarine

Fried foods

Commercially manufactured baked goods

Any food with partially hydrogenated oil
on its list of ingredients

Saturated fat: BAD. Saturated fats are naturally occurring fats found in meat and dairy products. The problem with saturated fats is that when they enter your body, they tend to do the same thing they did when they were in a pig's or cow's body: Rather than be burned for energy, they're more likely to be stored as fat in your flanks, in your ribs, even—ugh—in your loin. In fact, they seem to have more of a "storage effect" than other fats. A new study from Johns Hopkins University suggests that the amount of saturated fat in your diet may be directly proportional to the amount of fat surrounding your abdominal muscles. Researchers analyzed the diets of 84 people and performed an MRI on each of them to measure fat. Those whose diets included the highest rates of saturated fat also had the most abdominal fat. Saturated fats also raise cholesterol levels, so they increase your risk for heart disease and some types of cancer.

I don't want you to eliminate saturated fats entirely; they're found in most animal products, and those food products are important for the Abs Diet for other reasons (the calcium in dairy products, the protein in meat). But I do want you to consume the low-fat and leaner versions of meat and dairy products. You want the nutritional benefit from one part of the food without high amounts of saturated fat.

AVOID

Fatty cuts of red meat

Whole-milk dairy products

Polyunsaturated fats: GOOD. There are two types of polyunsaturated fats: omega-3s and omega-6s. You've probably heard of omega-3 fatty acids. They're the fats found in fish, and a diet high in omega-3s has been shown to help protect the heart from cardiovascular disease. That's plenty enough reason to include seafood in your diet. But new evidence suggests that this type of fat can actually help you control your weight. In one study, subjects who took in 6 grams a day of fish oil supplements burned more fat during the course of a day than those who went without. Researchers suspect that a diet high in omega-3s actually alters the body's metabolism and spurs it to burn fat more efficiently.

||||||||||||||||||||||||||||||||||||||||||||||||||||||||||||||||||||||||||||||||||||||||||||||||||

Seafood with the Highest Omega-3 Content

All data are for 3-ounce servings (except for sardines, which is for $3\frac{3}{4}$ ounces). Aim for a total of 2.5 grams (g) of omega-3s per day.

TYPE OF FISH	OMEGA-3 CONTENT (G)	PREPARED
Shad	3.7	Baked
Sardines	2.4	Water-packed can
Mackerel	1.9	Broiled
Sablefish	1.9	Broiled
Salmon	1.6	Poached
Tuna	1.5	Grilled
Oysters	1.4	Boiled
Trout	1.2	Broiled
Shark	1.1	Grilled
Swordfish	1.1	Grilled
Tuna, light	0.24	Water-packed can

Now, you can take fish oil supplements if you want, but you'll miss the lean, muscle-building protein benefits of real fish. The fish with the highest levels of omega-3s are the fish you probably enjoy the most already—salmon and tuna, to name two. (To see where your favorite fish falls in the omega-3 sweepstakes, see the chart on the opposite page.)

There's another amazing, secret powerfood that bodybuilders know about but you may have never even heard of: flaxseed. Flax is a seldom-used grain that's loaded with omega-3s as well as cholesterol-busting fiber. You'll find flaxseed and flaxseed oil in most health food stores. Grab it! I keep ground flaxseed in the fridge, and I toss it on breakfast cereals, into smoothies, and on top of ice cream. It's got a mild nutty flavor you'll like. It crushes cholesterol with its omega-3s, it adds artery-scouring fiber to your diet, and it might just be your best weapon against fat.

Omega-6 fatty acids also help lower bad cholesterol and raise good cholesterol. They're found in vegetable oils, meat, eggs, and dairy products. They're so common to so many foods, in fact, that only those of you currently shipwrecked on deserted islands living off flotsam and jetsam need worry about not getting enough in your diet.

EAT MORE

Fish

Flaxseed and flaxseed oil

Monounsaturated fats: GOOD. Monounsaturated fats are found in nuts, olives, peanuts, avocados, and olive and canola oils. Like omega-3s, these fats help reduce cholesterol levels and protect against heart disease, but they also help you burn fat; in one study, researchers found that the body burns more fat in the 5 hours following a meal high in monos than after a meal rich in saturated fats.

Monounsaturated fats will not only lower your cholesterol and help you burn off your belly but also help you eat less. Penn State researchers found that men who ate mashed potatoes prepared with oil high in monounsaturated fats like olive oil felt fuller longer than when they ate taters cooked with polyunsaturated fats like vegetable oil. And in another study, participants who ate bread with olive oil consumed nearly 25 percent less bread than they did when they ate bread slathered with butter, a saturated fat.

Carbohydrates: A Bad Rap

WITH THE BEATINGS that carbohydrates have taken over the past few years, it's a wonder that bread isn't protected by the Endangered Species Act. Everywhere I look, I see people eating burgers without buns, ordering spaghetti and meatballs—hold the spaghetti—or bragging about their all-bacon-all-the-time diet. While it's clear that protein and fat have tremendous nutritional benefits, it's unfair—and unhealthy—to kick carbohydrates off the dietary island.

With more and more evidence showing that a high-carbohydrate diet helps promote fat storage (unless you run marathons), it's becoming more accepted that low-carbohydrate diets work in helping people control weight. A 2002 study in the journal *Metabolism* confirmed that very stance. Researchers at the University of Connecticut found that subjects who ate only 46 grams of carbohydrates a day—about 8 percent of calories—lost 7 pounds of fat and gained 2 pounds of muscle in 6 weeks. And they did it while downing a satisfying 2,337 calories a day. But you can make a major mistake by eliminating carbohydrates entirely. Many carbohydrates—like fruits, vegetables, whole grains, and beans—help protect you against cancer and other diseases, and some carbs contain nutrients like fiber, which helps you lose and control weight.

Traditionally, the confusion about carbohydrates has centered around finding ways to classify them and figuring out which ones are better for your body. It used to be that we thought of carbohydrates only by their molecular structure—either simple or complex. Simple indicates a carb with one or two sugar molecules—things like sucrose (table sugar), fructose (in fruit), and lactose (in dairy products). Complex carbohydrates are ones that include more than two sugar molecules—like pasta, rice, bread, and potatoes. The flaw is that you can't generalize and say a carbohydrate is good or bad for you based simply on its molecular structure. For example, an apple contains nutrients and helps keep you lean; sugar does not. Both are simple carbs, but they're hardly comparable in nutritional value.

Instead, the way to decide what carbohydrates are best for you stems from how your body reacts to the carbohydrates chemically. One of the tools that nutritionists use today is the glycemic index (GI). The GI assigns numbers to foods that indicate how quickly a food turns into glucose. High-GI foods—ones that are quickly digested and turned to glucose—are generally less nutritionally sound than low-GI choices.

Another term for glucose is blood sugar. The presence of sugar in your blood causes your body to produce the hormone insulin. Insulin's job is to move the sugar you're not using for energy out of your bloodstream and store it in your body. Here's where the GI comes into effect: Foods with a high GI (like pasta, bread, white rice, and Snickers bars) are digested quickly, flooding your bloodstream with sugar. Insulin rushes in and says, "Whoa, what do I do with all of this?" Whatever glucose isn't immediately burned for energy quickly starts getting stored as fat. What's worse is that if you eat a carb with a high GI in combination with fat—bread with butter, for example—none of the fat you eat can be burned for energy either, because your bloodstream is so flooded with sugar. Insulin does such a good job of turning this new blood sugar into fat, in fact, that soon your blood sugar begins to drop, and you know what that means: You're hungry again.

If you eat a meal with a low GI (like a balanced dinner of chicken, high-fiber vegetables, and brown rice), the food is digested more slowly. Your blood sugar rises only incrementally, and that slow digestion means that glucose is available as energy for hours and hours. That means you have hours and hours to burn off the blood sugar. Insulin doesn't need to rush in and turn the sugar into fat; it can use the sugar slowly for other construction projects, like building and repairing muscle. Moreover, because your blood sugar levels stay even, you don't turn ravenously hungry just a few hours after eating. You build more muscle, you store less fat, you have more energy, and you keep your appetite under control.

(By the way, if all this talk about blood sugar and insulin reminds you of a certain health problem—diabetes—then you were obviously paying attention in health class. Continuing to flood your bloodstream with high levels of sugar, followed by high levels of insulin, eventually trains your body to become less efficient at processing these blood sugars. That's called insulin resistance, which is another term for diabetes. It is a terrible, terrible disease—and it is also highly preventable. In a Harvard study, men who ate foods with the lowest GIs, like whole-wheat bread, were 37 percent less likely to develop diabetes than those who ate high-GI foods, such as white rice. (For more information on battling diabetes, see our Health Bulletin on page 54.)

It's hard to generalize about which carbs are high on the GI list and which are low, because glycemic index is simply a measure of time—that is, how long it takes 50 grams of the food's carbohydrates to turn into blood sugar, regardless of serving size. It's a measure, for instance, of the carb-to-sugar conversion time for a whole apple or watermelon, but it doesn't tell you how much carb is in one serving of the food. Nobody eats a whole watermelon, anyway.

That's why the latest advancement in food science is to look at a meal's glycemic load (GL). The GL considers both the GI of a food and the amount of carbs in one serving of that food. It helps you gauge the glycemic effect, or the projected elevation of blood glucose, that food will cause.

The higher a food's GL, the more it will cause your blood sugar to spike, and the less control you'll have over your energy and appetite. But considering the GL is only one aspect of creating a balanced diet. "It's better to have a high-GL diet than one full of saturated fat," says Jennie Brand-Miller, PhD, professor of human nutrition at the University of Sydney and author of the *International Table of Glycemic Index and Glycemic Load*. "Aiming for the lowest GL possible is not a good move because that means you'll be eating too little carbohydrate and too much fat—probably saturated fat." Instead, to maintain your body's best glycemic response, center your meals around foods with GLs of 19 or less and shoot for a GL of less than 120 for the whole day.

Sound confusing? It doesn't need to be. The 12 Abs Diet Powerfoods and the Abs Diet recipes all have low to moderate glycemic loads. All you have to do is follow the plan. And on those occasions when you are stuck and need to choose between two or more foods, refer to the chart on page 298.

Calcium: The Future of Fat Fighting

YOU'VE SEEN MORE than enough milk mustaches to know that calcium strengthens your bones, but did you know that calcium can also firm up your gut? Researchers at Harvard Medical School showed that those who ate three servings of dairy a day—which in conjunction with other foods provides about 1,200 milligrams of calcium (about the daily recommendation)—were 60 percent less likely to be overweight. In studies at the University of Tennessee, researchers put subjects on diets that were 500 calories a day less than what they were used to eating. Yup, the subjects lost weight—about 1 pound of fat a week. But when researchers put another set of subjects on the same diet but added dairy to their meals, their fat loss doubled, to 2 pounds a week. Same calorie intake, double the fat loss.

Calcium seems to limit the amount of new fat your body can make, according to the University of Tennessee research team. In another study conducted at the same lab, men who added three servings of yogurt a day to their diets lost 61 percent more body fat and 81 percent more stomach fat in 12 weeks than men who didn't eat yogurt. A study in Hawaii found that teens with the highest calcium intakes were thinner and leaner than those getting less calcium.

Some researchers speculate that dairy calcium helps fight fat because it increases the thermic effect of eating—in other words, you burn more calories digesting calcium-rich foods than you would if you ate something with equal calories but no calcium. That's one reason why calcium supplements, though good for bone-building and other bodily functions, don't have the same effect as dairy—fewer calories to digest, so fewer calories to burn.

And calcium has its benefits beyond stronger bones and leaner bodies. After analyzing data from 47,000 men involved in the Health Professional's Follow-Up Study, Harvard researchers found that men whose diets included 700 to 800 milligrams of the mineral a day were up to 50 percent less likely to develop some forms of colon cancer than men whose diets contained less than 500 milligrams. For best effect, shoot for about 1,200 milligrams (mg) of calcium per day.

The New Abs Diet recommended calcium-rich foods are:

▶ 1 ounce grated Parmesan cheese (314 mg)

▶ 1 cup large-curd cottage cheese (126 mg)

▶ 8 ounces low-fat yogurt (415 mg)

▶ 8 ounces low-fat milk (340 mg)

▶ 1 ounce (1-inch cube) Swiss cheese (224 mg)

▶ 1 ounce (1 slice) Cheddar cheese (204 mg)

▶ 1 ounce mozzarella cheese (143 mg)

▶ 1 scoop (28 g) whey powder protein (110 mg)

Chapter 5

A SIX-PACK IN 6 WEEKS
A Week-by-Week Guide to How Your Body Will Change

I F YOU FLIP THROUGH THIS book, you'll meet some of the men and women who went on the Abs Diet—and succeeded. Patrick Austin dropped 30 pounds, half of it in just the first 2 weeks. Now he can't wait to take off his shirt at the beach.

John Betson turned a flabby 36-inch waist into a solid 32-incher and saw his abs for the first time in years.

Jessica Guff stopped skipping meals—and started wearing skimpy tops.

For Bill Stanton, the turnaround was an eye-opener: "I'd been lifting weights all my life, but just by changing my diet, my body got leaner and stronger than ever. Guys at the gym even accuse me of being on steroids!"

Everyone's body is different, and everybody who tries this plan will have a different starting point. But based on the scientific research I've outlined, you can expect an average loss of up to 20 pounds of fat on the 6-week plan and, for men, a gain of 4 to 6 pounds of muscle (about half that amount for women). For the average man, that's enough of a transformation to have your abs show. One of the bigger challenges, however, is monitoring your progress on the plan.

Here's a look at the four major measurements you can use to see just how effectively the New Abs Diet will work for you.

Weight. It's the most straightforward. The heavier you are, the more at risk you are for disease and the less fit you are. It's a good measuring stick to gauge how well you're progressing on your diet, but it's incomplete in that it doesn't take into account the amount of muscle you're going to develop over the course of a plan. Muscle weighs about 20 percent more than fat so even a dramatic fat loss may not translate into a dramatic drop in body weight.

Body mass index (BMI). The BMI is a formula that takes into consideration your height and your weight, and gives you an indication of whether you're overweight, obese, or in good shape. To calculate your BMI, multiply your weight in pounds by 703, and divide the number by your height in inches squared. For example, let's say you are 6 feet tall (that's 72 inches) and weigh 200 pounds. So first we multiply your weight by 703.

||||||||||||||||||||||||||||||||||||||||||||||||||||||||||||||||||||||||||||||||||||||||||||||||||||

Insulin: The Two-Faced Hormone

The hormone insulin is like your pack-rat grandmother: It likes to store stuff. The only problem is that it's also as schizophrenic as old Uncle Judd. Sometimes it makes your muscles grow; sometimes it makes your fat cells grow.

Different foods create different insulin responses. Foods that have high–glycemic index rankings (including white bread, most cereals, grapes, and bananas) dump a lot of sugar into your bloodstream soon after eating, causing insulin levels to spike. In this case, insulin works quickly to turn that blood sugar into fat.

Some foods, though, cause a different reaction. Dairy products—milk, yogurt, ice cream—create dramatic insulin surges without the corresponding effect on blood sugar. You also get this insulin response from some foods that are virtually carbohydrate-free, such as beef and fish, which have hardly any effect on blood sugar. When blood sugar remains relatively constant, it allows insulin to use the nutrients in your blood to build and repair cells, including muscle tissue.

That's why the Abs Diet centers around high-fiber, nutrient-dense foods that are also the ones thought to be most useful for weight control. Most are moderate to high protein, some are high in dairy calcium, and those that are carb-based emphasize fiber and other important nutrients.

200 × 703 = 140,600

Next, we calculate your height in inches squared, meaning we multiply the number by itself.

72 × 72 = 5,184

Now we divide the first number by the second.

140,600 ÷ 5,184 = 27.1

That's not terrible. A BMI between 25 and 30 indicates you're overweight. Over 30 signifies obesity.

This measurement, too, has flaws. It doesn't take into account muscle mass, and it also leaves out another important factor—weight distribution, that is, where most of the fat on your body resides. But BMI can give you a pretty good idea of how serious your weight problem is.

Waist-to-hip ratio. Researchers have begun using waist size and its relationship to hip size as a more definitive way to determine your health risk. This is considered more important than BMI because of that visceral fat I talked about earlier—the fat that pushes your waist out in front of you. Because abdominal fat is the most dangerous fat, a lower waist-to-hip ratio means fewer health risks. To figure out your waist-to-hip ratio, measure your waist at your belly button and your hips at the widest point (around your butt). Divide your waist by your hips. For example, if your hips measure 40 inches and your waist at belly button level measures 38 inches, your waist-to-hip ratio is 0.95.

38 ÷ 40 = 0.95

That's not bad, but it's not ideal. You want a waist-to-hip ratio of 0.92 or lower. If you were to lose just 2 inches off your waist—something you can do in just 2 weeks with the Abs Diet—you'd find yourself in the fit range.

36 ÷ 40 = 0.90

Body fat percentage. Though this is the most difficult for the average person to measure because it requires a bit of technology, it's the most useful in terms of gauging how well your diet plan is working. That's because it takes into consideration not just weight but how much of your weight is fat.

Many gyms offer body fat measurements through such methods as body fat scales or calipers that measure the folds of fat at several points on your body. See your local gym for what options they offer. Or try an at-home body fat calculator. I like the Taylor Body Fat Analyzer and Scale 5553 for its price (about $50), convenience, and accuracy. If you want a simple low-tech test (and this isn't as accurate as what the electronic versions will give you), try this simple exercise: Sit in a chair with your knees bent and your feet flat on the floor. Using your thumb and index finger, gently pinch the skin on top of your right thigh. Measure the thickness of the pinched skin with a ruler. If it's ¾ inch or less, you have about 14 percent body fat—ideal for a guy, quite fit for a woman. It it's 1 inch, you're probably closer to 18 percent fat, which is a tad high for a man but desirable for a woman. If you pinch more than an inch, you could be at increased risk for diabetes and heart disease.

This last measurement can be the most significant because it'll really help give you a sense of how well you're sticking to a plan. As you see your body fat percentage decrease, you'll see an increase in the amount of visible muscle. Experts say that in order for your abs to show, your body fat needs to be between 8 and 12 percent. For the average slightly overweight man, that means cutting body fat by about half.

Before you start the plan, record some of these measurements so that you'll know how far you're progressing. Take one baseline measurement, and then remeasure as needed for motivation. I'd recommend measuring every 2 weeks. That'll be enough time to see significant differences to propel you through the next 2 weeks. (Measure body fat percentage only at the beginning and end of the plan, unless you have easy access to a measurement system.) Any sooner than that, and you're focusing too much on numbers rather than process.

MEASUREMENT	START	WEEK 2	WEEK 4	WEEK 6
Weight				
BMI				
Waist-to-hip ratio				
Body fat percentage*				

*Make sure to have the same person administer body fat readings using the same method to ensure consistency.

As with any diet plan, it's also important to develop some kind of quantitative goal—your ideal weight, waist size, or percentage of body fat. This chart will help you figure out where you are and where you need to go.

I don't mean to hit you with more numbers than a fantasy baseball nerd. In fact, it might be easiest to simply focus on one number—six—so that the others will fall into place. When you start to see those six abdominal muscles, it'll mean that everything else has decreased—your weight, your BMI, your waist-to-hip ratio, and your body fat percentage. This 6-week plan will get you there. Here's what you can expect from going on the diet.

WEEKS	WHAT TO EXPECT	WHAT THEY SAY
1-2	A significant weight loss as your body adjusts to a new approach to eating. Some may see losses up to 12 pounds in the first 2 weeks (especially if you're walking, or otherwise active, each day), but 5–8 pounds will be average	**PATRICK AUSTIN LOST 15 POUNDS IN JUST THE FIRST COUPLE OF WEEKS ON THE ABS DIET.** *"I haven't gone shirtless on the beach in years," he says. "This year, I'm going to be shirtless." Read more about Patrick's success on page 78.*
3-4	By integrating a modest amount of strength training into your routine, you'll start to feel your body change because your metabolism is working hard. You'll notice an additional drop in weight (most likely averaging another 5–8 pounds), but you'll also notice significant changes in your shape.	**BRIAN ARCHIQUETTE DROPPED 25 POUNDS IN 6 WEEKS.** *"I definitely have more energy and a more positive outlook on life," he says. Read more about Brian's success on page 168.*

WEEKS	WHAT TO EXPECT	WHAT THEY SAY
5-6	After 2 weeks of exercise, your body is primed to make a significant push to drop more fat while also gaining muscle mass. You'll notice that your upper body is more toned and that your waist and other fatty parts of your body are smaller. Depending on your starting point, this is where you'll begin to see abs.	**JOHN BETSON DECREASED HIS BODY FAT FROM 23 PERCENT TO 16 PERCENT.** *"You can see more muscle," he exclaims. "You can see my abs." Read more about John's success on page 134.*

What you'll find so remarkable about this program is how simple it is to follow, how often you'll eat—each meal and each snack is an easy, muscle-building, fat-burning treat—and how unlike any other "diet" the New Abs Diet is. Very simply, the New Abs Diet is a plan that will ask you to:

▶ Eat three meals and three snacks each day, with each of your meals or snacks including several of the wide-ranging powerfoods discussed in Chapter 8.

ABS DIET SUCCESS STORY

"I Cut My Body Fat in Half!"

Name: James Schellman

Age: 26

Height: 5'8"

Starting weight: 164

Six weeks later: 156

A former professional athlete and an active guy who snowboards 60 days a year, James Schellman didn't feel like he needed to lose that much weight. But then a series of nagging injuries started hampering his active lifestyle, and he packed on an extra 10 pounds of belly flab. Schellman could have blamed the weight gain and injuries on getting older, but that wasn't his style. "I didn't want to slow down," he says, "but I knew I needed a change." So he went on the Abs Diet to improve his condition and increase his muscle tone.

► Keep an eye out for a handful of diet busters that you'll learn to easily spot and cut down on—not eliminate.

► Perform a simple, 20-minute workout three times a week to turbo-charge your fat loss and muscle growth.

The New Abs Diet is so simple that, unlike most other diets, we don't break it into phases, and we didn't design a complex "maintenance" program (just a few simple words of wisdom that you'll find on page 283). The weight loss and muscle gains are yours to keep for life, and so is the eating plan. We guarantee you won't be waiting for your "diet" to end. You'll enjoy this program so much—and be so wowed by the results—that you'll effortlessly follow this plan for life.

Other people have done it—other people who were much heavier and in worse physical condition than you. When they talk about why the Abs Diet worked so effectively for them, they speak of the plan's simplicity and its ability to keep hunger in check. You'll see, too. The New Abs Diet is going to change your shape, your health, your life.

Besides, Schellman says, "I figured I need to look good for my wife."

During the plan, Schellman lost 8 pounds. But the most significant transformation: He cut his body fat from 18 to 11 percent.

Schellman has always enjoyed eating healthfully, but adjusting to the Abs Diet paid off. "Before the plan, I ate about four meals a day and counted calories. And with this one, I ate six times a day and let calories go by the wayside," he says. By basing meals around the delicious powerfoods, "I didn't have to worry about the calories I was taking in."

Schellman, who is used to spending a lot of time in the gym, credits the New Abs Diet Workout and its emphasis on lower-body exercises for making him stronger and leaner and helping him burn off that burgeoning belly. "I have seen stomach fat decrease. I can clearly see some of the muscles [in my abdomen]," he says. "The plan has been a huge success—I've seen an increase in my overall body strength, an increase in my motivation, an increase in my self-esteem, and an increase in my well-being."

ABS DIET HEALTH BULLETIN

What the Heck Are . . . Cancer Cells?

Cancer is the one scourge that can strike any of us at any time in life. It can hit in the places we think about and care about on a daily basis—the skin, the lungs, the brain—or in obscure places we don't even understand, like the pancreas, the kidneys, or the lymphatic system.

Simply put, cancer develops when cells in one part of the body begin to grow out of control. As children, our cells are constantly dividing, creating the new cells that help us grow. Once we reach adulthood, that cell growth stops, for the most part. Once we reach our genetically programmed height and weight, cells in most parts of the body divide only to replace worn-out or dying cells or to repair injuries. (That's why there's no mid-thirties growth spurt, much as we may wish for it.)

But cancer cells act like kids—they keep growing, dividing, and multiplying, outliving our normal cells and interfering with the various functions of the body. The most common type of cancer among men is prostate cancer (the prostate is the gland located behind the scrotum that produces most of our seminal fluid). The most common type of cancer among women is breast cancer. Both result in about a quarter million new cases every year.

We don't fully understand what causes cancer, but we do know some of the risk factors: Obesity, low-fiber diets, smoking, heavy alcohol use, overexposure to the sun, and exposure to radiation and other toxins are among the biggest dangers. Additionally, there's a strong link between heredity and cancer. If one or more close relatives has suffered a bout of the disease, you're at increased risk for cancer in general and for that specific form of cancer in particular.

I'd like to tell you that the New Abs Diet is a magic bullet against cancer, but I can't. While dietary changes and exercise can dramatically decrease your risk for heart disease, stroke, and especially diabetes, cancer remains a bit more elusive. Still, by adopting the principles of the New Abs Diet, you'll automatically decrease your risk for many forms of cancer, because you'll decrease your weight and increase your fiber intake. In the meantime, you can also follow these additional tips to slash your risk even more:

Toss in the tomatoes. Tomatoes are one of the best sources of lycopene, a nutrient that has been shown to inhibit the growth of prostate cancer cells. In fact, researchers say that two to four servings of tomatoes a week can cut your prostate cancer risk by 34 percent. (Even better news: Lycopene isn't diminished by cooking, so pasta sauce and pizza will strike a blow against the disease as well.)

Go for yolk. Research in 2009 suggests that egg yolk may be cancer-protective. The yellow stuff is rich in choline, which has been linked to lower rates of breast cancer. One yolk delivers 25 percent of your daily needs.

Hail a cabbage. Each 22-calorie cup of cabbage is loaded with sulforaphane, a chemical that increases your body's production of the enzymes that disarm cell-damaging, cancer-causing free radicals.

Be like Popeye. A 2009 report in the *International Journal of Cancer* shows that people who ate the most folate-rich leafy greens, such as spinach, had half as many skin cancer tumors as those who ate the least. It's thought that the folate in greens like spinach may help repair DNA.

Color your plate. A 14-year study found that men whose diets were highest in fruits and vegetables had a 70 percent lower risk of digestive-tract cancers.

Order the Chilean red. Chilean cabernet sauvignon is 38 percent higher than French wine in flavonols—compounds called antioxidants that help deter cancer.

Try the cheese platter. A large-scale study of 120,000 women found that premenopausal women who consumed a lot of dairy products, especially low-fat and fat-free ones, ran a lower risk of breast cancer. Pay attention, men: You can get breast cancer, too. And Harvard researchers have found that men with diets high in calcium were up to 50 percent less likely to develop some forms of colon cancer.

Bite the broccoli. It contains a compound called indole-3-carbinol, which has been shown to fight various forms of cancer. Don't like broccoli? Try daikon, an Asian radish that looks like a big white carrot. It's a distant cousin.

Serve the salmon. Or any other fish high in omega-3 fatty acids. Omega-3s can help mollify your cancer risk.

Go green. In a recent Rutgers University study, mice given green tea had 51 percent fewer incidences of skin cancer than control mice. Green tea is another great source of cancer-fighting antioxidants.

Get a D. Foods high in vitamin D, like low-fat milk, help detoxify cancer-causing chemicals released during the digestion of high-fat foods, according to a study at the University of Texas Southwestern Medical Center.

Show yourself the whey. Whey protein is a great source of cysteine, a major building block of the prostate cancer–fighting agent glutathione.

Eat the whole grain. Whole-grain carbohydrates are a great source of fiber. European researchers found that men with the highest daily intakes of fiber also had a 40 percent lower risk of developing colon cancer.

Chapter 6

SHOCKER: HOW LOW-CARB DIETS MAKE YOU FAT

The Truth about the Trend That's Threatening America's Health

THROUGHOUT THIS BOOK, I've hit you with scientific evidence, persuaded you with real-life testimonials, and referenced study after study to show how the Abs Diet works and why it makes sense for anyone who wants to manage his weight and live a healthful, active, disease-free life. But just for a moment, I want to step away from all the hard science and take you on a bit of a fantasy adventure. Come this way—I promise you'll find it revealing.

First, I want you to imagine that you've taken a time machine back to the Middle Ages. You find yourself at the door of an alchemist's laboratory, where magic elixirs and potions fill the shelves and the echoes of mantras and spells fill the air. You've traveled long and hard, through terrifying dark woods and vast, arid deserts to seek out a Holy Grail of sorts: a concoction that legend says will make you lose weight, magically.

The sorcerer appears, and he holds up before you two vials. The first, he says, contains an elixir that will protect you from most of the diseases known to man. Its ingredients hold properties that will change your cholesterol profile and protect you from heart disease; help scour your body for toxins and protect you from the onslaught of cancer and the side effects of aging; energize your body and your brain, making your thinking clearer and helping to immunize you from Alzheimer's; and, over the course of your long life, control your weight and keep obesity and diabetes at bay.

The second vial will do none of that. It will, in all likelihood, raise your cholesterol profile and increase your risk for cancer, stroke, and heart disease, as well as other ailments. But, if you take it, it may help you lose weight dramatically—though only for a short period of time. And there's one more drawback: If you choose the second vial, you can never sip from the first.

Which do you choose?

In the past 10 years, more than 60 million Americans chose vial number two.

Now, scrape the dust from the label on that vial and guess what it says? Low-carbohydrate diet.

ABS DIET SUCCESS STORY

"I Deflated My Spare Tire!"

Name: Patrick Austin

Age: 33

Height: 6'

Starting weight: 245

Six weeks later: 215

Patrick Austin thought he had the perfect solution for his spare tire. At 6 feet and 245 pounds, and several years removed from high school football, Austin had decided to take his fitness into his own hands. He hired a personal trainer and started to attack the fat.

But after 6 months of working one-on-one, nothing happened. "I don't think the personal trainer personalized the program for me," Austin says. "I think he used a general plan he used for everybody. There was no push."

Then Austin stumbled across the Abs Diet and tried it. Within 10 days of his starting the Abs Diet, people in the gym were asking

The first vial, on the other hand, brims with all sorts of things: fruits and vegetables, whole-grain breads and cereals, beans and nuts—the sorts of things that nature intended us to eat but diet plans like Atkins's do not. And over the long term, if Americans keep choosing vial number two, I think we're going to pay—heavily.

The Origins of a Sweet Tooth

TO UNDERSTAND WHY carbohydrates are important, we have to take another fantasy trip, this time back to the dawn of man. On the savannahs of Africa, the high plains of Europe, the wetlands of Asia, and the woodlands and jungles of the Americas, primitive man learned how to feed himself from nature's banquet table. He learned how to fish and hunt, and later, how to domesticate animals and grow grain. But since he first stood upright, man has also had a craving for sweets.

him what he'd been doing differently. He lost 15 pounds within the first couple of weeks, and he attributes it to a change in his approach to eating.

"I'm not the kind of person who eats a lot, but I was eating the wrong kinds of food," Austin says. "When I tried to lose weight before, I'd always watch my calories. But with the Abs Diet, you eat many meals—but concentrate on the right kinds of food."

So instead of indulgences of cakes, pies, and pastries after every meal, Austin downed smoothies, lean meats, and eggs. "Almonds became my best friend. They carry me over when I'm hungry in between meals."

Austin also stayed dedicated to the workout—lifting weights 3 days a week and doing some type of cardio work on 3 other days.

Though he feels the best he's felt in years, Austin says he has one more goal. Every year, he and his wife go on a beach vacation with some other couples.

"I'm fanatical about the water. I love the pool. I love the beach. But I haven't gone shirtless on the beach in years. That's my goal this year," Austin says. "When we go this year, I'm going to be shirtless."

As with all things, there's a reason why we crave sweets. The sweetest things on earth, back in those days before Cherry Garcia, were fruits: wild berries, pears, citrus fruits, and the like. Not coincidentally, fruits are also packed with nutrients: vitamins to fend off disease; minerals to assist with cell function; and fiber to regulate hunger, control blood pressure, and help ease digestion. Without our sweet tooth, we would have been happy to eat nothing but woolly mammoth and buffalo meat—the original Atkins program. But nature saw to it that we craved the foods that would make us healthy.

Fast forward to today, when the sweetest things don't look anything like tangerines. Whereas our sweet tooth was once nature's way of protecting us from disease, now it's the food industry's way of tricking us into it. To satisfy our cravings, we turn to cookies and cakes and chocolates instead of apples and pears and blackberries. That's one of the main reasons Americans today are so fat. And it's one of the main reasons why, in the short-term, low-carb diets work.

By limiting carbohydrate intake, diets like Atkins create by-default weight loss. If you restrict yourself to just one class of foods—low-carb foods, in this instance—you're bound to lose weight. That's because the stuff you're used to munching on, from the doughnut you nosh in the car on the way to work to the Snickers bar you snag from the vending machine before your drive home, are now voided from your diet. You're eating less food, so you're taking in fewer calories, so you lose weight.

The other sneaky advantage of an Atkins diet is that it focuses on foods that are difficult to prepare and consume. It's easy to pop a bagel or a grapefruit into your briefcase; shove some steak and eggs in there instead, and things get a little messy. So low-carb diets restrict calories in two ways: by limiting food options, and by limiting the ease with which we can consume food.

But there are two major reasons why, in the long-term, low-carb diets won't work: Mother Nature and the almighty dollar.

Low-Carb Dilemma #1: Take That Out of Your Mouth!

SOMEONE WITH A sound understanding of nutrition and a sadistic streak could have a field day torturing low-carb enthusiasts. Here's an evil trick: Take two pieces of soft, fresh, whole-grain bread. Slather one side with 2 tablespoons of all-natural peanut butter. Now take ½ cup of blackberries, mash them lightly with a fork, and (this is where it gets really nasty) spread the mashed berries onto the other piece of bread. Put the two sides together and you've created the world's healthiest PB&J sandwich: 5 grams of fiber (about as much as the average American gets in a single day), 25 percent of your daily intake of vitamin C, 13 grams of protein, and (sacre bleu!) a verboten 30 grams of carbohydrate. (Oh, by the way, it tastes incredible.)

Float this concoction in front of a low-carb enthusiast and you might as well be serving broiled rat viscera. (Come to think of it, they'd probably prefer the rat viscera. No carbs.) The sandwich is achingly sweet, soft, and chewy—a delicious comfort food that, at the same time, is a cholesterol-busting nuclear missile. The fiber protects you from heart disease as well as from stroke and colon cancer. The vitamin C boosts your immune system. And the high-quality (meaning high in fiber) carbs give you long-burning energy and food for your brain. Yet phase one of the Atkins diet bans every single ingredient in this simple sandwich.

Every single one.

In fact, the Atkins diet focuses on something called net carbs that Atkins claims are the carbohydrates that actually impact blood sugar. A rough formula for figuring out net carbs is to subtract the number of fiber grams from the total number of carb grams. (The reasoning being that fiber doesn't impact blood sugar, spike insulin, or contribute to fat storage.) By that calculation, this sandwich has about 33 net carbs. Phase one of the Atkins diet limits you to 20 net carbs per day. Eat this one super-good-for-you food, and you'll have to fast for the next day and a half to keep your Atkins diet in effect.

Maybe it's just me, but I think this whole low-carb plan is simply crackers. (Oh, sorry—not allowed to eat those.)

See, carbs are not our enemies. As I explained earlier, we crave carbs because we need them to protect us against a host of ailments. The low-carb craze works temporarily not because it limits carbs but because it limits food intake. And if I came out with some crazy diet plan that said you could only eat foods that are high in fat or low in protein or bigger than a breadbox or start with the letter P, believe me—you'd lose weight. For a little while, at least, until you couldn't look at pudding, parsnips, and poultry ever again.

You'd lose weight because, by restricting your food intake, I've restricted your calorie intake. And the fact is, when you take in fewer calories than you burn, you lose weight; when you take in more calories than you burn, you gain weight. That's true regardless of where those calories come from. The New Abs Diet works both by cutting the number of calories you take in through a sensible-but-satiating eating plan and by increasing the number of calories you burn away by improving your metabolic function. Fewer calories coming in here, a few more burned off there, and presto—weight loss. No magic, no deprivation, and no pointing fingers at the evils of carbohydrates.

The confusion about carbs comes from the fact that, in today's society, we're surrounded by high-carbohydrate foods that have had all their positive attributes stripped from them. The refined flours and sugars and sugar substitutes that you find in everything from cookies to ice cream to mass-produced ketchup and peanut butter give us all the calories and none of the nutritional benefits of their original ancestors: whole grains and fruits. The lack of fiber in, say, a plain bagel causes the calories in the bagel to be digested quickly, flooding our bloodstreams with glucose, triggering spikes in the digestive hormone insulin—which then turns the blood sugar into fat cells and leaves us hungry once again.

But fruits, vegetables, and whole-grain bread products have a very different effect on the body: They're digested slowly, giving us long-burning energy. Insulin levels stay steady while fiber scours our bodies for cholesterol and other harmful substances, and the vitamins and minerals inherent in those foods help protect us from a host of ills.

||||||||||||||||||||||||||||||||||||||||||||||||||||||||||||||||||||||||||||||||||||||||||||||||||||||

Five Ways to Add More Fiber

To your eggs: A third of a cup of chopped onion and a clove of garlic will add 1 gram of fiber to a couple of scrambled eggs.

To your sandwich: Hate whole wheat? Go with rye. Like wheat, it has 2 grams of fiber per slice. That's more than twice the amount of fiber in white.

To your dinner: Have a sweet potato. It has 2 grams more fiber than a typical Idaho potato.

To your cereal: Half a cup of raspberries adds 4 grams of fiber.

To your snack: Eat trail mix. Half a cup of Raisin Bran, 1 ounce of mixed nuts, and five dried apricot halves give you almost 7 grams of fiber.

The longer we try to go without carbs, the more our bodies crave them. Eventually, you have to fall off a carb-restricting diet: Your body is programmed to make you seek out carbs, just the way it's programmed to blink when something hurtles toward your eye. It's one of our natural defense mechanisms, and what Mother Nature wants, she will eventually get.

Then again, what corporate America wants, it too will get. Which presents us with part two of why the low-carb craze is a disaster waiting to happen.

Low-Carb Dilemma #2: Follow the Money

REMEMBER WHAT I said about why the low-carb diet appears to work? Because it cuts out a majority of foods that people love to eat, and because it makes eating on the run difficult. Those two factors conspire to restrict calories, and fewer calories mean less weight.

Now, here's an easy question: How do food manufacturers make money? By selling you food. So what happens when 60 million Americans decide they're going to stop buying all the candy bars, loaves of bread, boxes of pasta, and jars of sugary spreads that manufacturers have obligingly loaded with carbohydrates over the past half century?

Food manufacturers are going to have to come up with something else to sell. Something they can tout as low carb, to appeal to Atkins-oriented dieters, but something that's familiar, easy to find, and even easier to consume. And so begins the next phase in the American obesity epidemic.

In February 2004, the *New York Times* reported on the growing trend toward low-carb marketing among restaurants and grocery stores. Retailers were being counseled by their business advisors to open up "low-carb" aisles; restaurants were vying for the coveted "Atkins approved" label to hang in their windows. And in the past 6 years, nearly 1,000 new food products claiming to be low in carbohydrates have hit the shelves. Today, you can snack on low-carb candy, low-carb cake, and low-carb brownies, washing it all down with a couple bottles of low-carb beer.

To get a sneak preview of where all this is going, let's hop back into that time travel machine. This time, we're not going to the storied Middle Ages or the dawn of man . . . we're just going back about 17 years or so, to the beginnings of the last diet craze that swept the nation: the low-fat craze.

It's the early 1990s. The low-carb craze hasn't yet begun to blossom. (For better or worse, neither has Britney Spears.) But another mantra has begun to take hold in American society: Eat less fat.

This directive comes not from a book-peddling diet doc but from the US government, in the form of a revised food pyramid designed by the Food and Drug Administration. Fat has been fingered as the root of all dietary evils: Simply put, fatty foods translate into fatty people. Diet experts race to defend this idea, which on the face of it sounds pretty logical: Dietary fat is more easily transformed into body fat, whereas carbohydrates are preferentially burned off for energy. Hence, swap your fat calories for carb calories, and voilà, you've entered into the magical weight loss zone.

Quickly, food manufacturers move to capitalize on these exciting developments. As sales of fat-free milk rise, packages of reduced-fat, low-fat, and fat-free cheeses, spreads, yogurts, ice creams, cakes, and cookies begin to fill the supermarket shelves. Some taste okay. Some taste like sugar-crusted cardboard. But what the hell—no fat, no foul. Carbo-loading becomes a byword of amateur athletes all across the country.

However, this whole low-fat theory comes with one big but. (Actually, it comes with millions of big butts, as the obesity rate has risen 15 percent in the past 10 years.) Like today's low-carb craze, the low-fat craze originally appears to work because it creates a restrictive eating program that eliminates certain foods and, hence, a certain number of calories. If you suddenly have to cut out countless steaks, baked goods, slabs of butter, nuts, dairy products, and desserts, presto, you lose weight.

But, as with carbohydrates, our bodies crave fat. Fatty foods (beef, fish, and dairy products, for instance) are usually high in muscle-building proteins and supply critical vitamins and minerals (the vitamin E in nuts and oils, the calcium in cheese and yogurt). So you can go on a low-fat diet for only so long before you wind up facedown in a pint of Chunky Monkey. That's the way Mother Nature planned it.

What she didn't plan for, however, was the craftiness of food marketers. Knowing that low-fat dieters are secretly pining for a nice slice of cake and a scoop of ice cream, grocery manufacturers go into the laboratory and come out with hundreds of new low-fat foods. And that leads to what should go down in history as The Great SnackWell's Debacle.

Nabisco conceives SnackWell's as the ultimate answer to the low-fat diet craze. SnackWell's, which you can still find on grocery shelves today, are fat-free and low-fat cookies that somehow carry nearly all the flavor of full-fat cookies. The secret is that Nabisco loads up the cookies with extra sugar (except in the sugar-free varieties), so consumers can indulge their sweet tooth without ever missing the fat. How this development plays out in the mind of the average consumer is simple to predict:

"All I have to do to lose weight is to cut out fat."

"Yo! These cookies have no fat. Let's buy two packages!"

"Honey, did you eat that second package of cookies for breakfast? I wanted it!"

The magic bullet doesn't work, in part because we need to eat fats and in part because we've been fooled into thinking that we can eat whatever we want, in whatever quantity we want, as long as we aren't eating fat. So we scarf down sugar calories by the spoonful—and we all get just a little bit fatter in the process.

Okay, hop out of the time machine—trip's over. It's a decade later and, instead of a low-fat craze, America is caught up in the throes of a low-carb craze. And the same scenario is playing out all over again. Every grocery store and corner deli is filled with products—particularly "meal replacement" bars—that are marketed with bywords like low-carb or carb smart.

Suddenly, it's not hard to eat low-carb anymore. Today—and increasingly so tomorrow—we can fill our shopping carts with all the foods we cut out for the past couple of years. Food marketers are altering the makeups of their products, packing them with soy protein and fiber and sugar alcohols—all ingredients that lower the "net carb" impact of the food. Now, I'm all for more protein and fiber. Sugar alcohol, on the other hand, is nothing but empty calories that, in elevated quantities, cause gastric distress and flatulence—but hey, whatever turns you on.

What I am against is the notion that marketers are peddling—that we can eat whatever and whenever we want, as long as we're not eating carbs. It is exactly the same trap we fell into more than 10 years ago: a restrictive diet that offers short-term success, turned into a food craze that guarantees even greater health risks and higher obesity rates.

And that's a time travel destination no one wants to arrive at.

Chapter 7

THE NEW ABS DIET NUTRITION PLAN

The Powerfoods and System That
Will Change Your Body

E ARLIER IN THE BOOK,
I gave an overview of some cool science—how your body reacts to different foods, why some fats are good and others are evil, and how some foods such as dairy products have a secret ingredient that helps your body burn fat. Science can be fun, but by this point in the book, you've probably got one burning question in your mind:

Hey, when can we eat?

So let's get right to it, because eating more of the right foods more often is the basis of the New Abs Diet. Remember:

MORE FOOD = MORE MUSCLE = LESS FLAB

That's why the New Abs Diet isn't a diet you'll feel you "have to" stick to. It's one you'll want to stick to.

See, I've talked to lots of people who've tried diets, and many of them describe trying to stick to a strict diet plan as sort of like standing waist-deep in the ocean and being pummeled by one wave after another. Those waves come in the form of doughnuts the boss brought in, the office vending machine you're stuck with when the boss makes you work late, and the happy hour to celebrate the firing of the boss who gave you all those doughnuts and late vending machine nights. When you're staring at a wave that's clearly bigger than you, you have three choices. You could run back to shore or try to jump over it, but those options will leave you with a suit full of sand. But if you dive through the wave head-on, you'll emerge unscathed. Same with a diet. You can try to run away by avoiding restaurants, parties, weddings, or anyplace that's likely to tempt you with nachos grande. You can also try to take the high road, but ordering a salad and water after a softball game hardly feels right. If you want a diet to work—if you want to emerge on the other side of this plan with a new body—your only choice is to have the flexibility and freedom to keep yourself from getting hungry and the knowledge that you can eat well no matter what.

You're about to dive into the New Abs Diet.

Guideline 1: Eat Six Meals a Day

WE'RE SO USED to hearing people talk about eating less food that it's become weight-loss doctrine. But as you remember from the physiology of metabolism, you have to eat more often to change your body composition. The new philosophy I want you to keep in mind is "energy balance."

Researchers at Georgia State University developed a technique to measure hourly energy balance—that is, how many calories you're burning versus how many calories you're taking in. The researchers found that if you keep your hourly surplus or deficit within 300 to 500 calories at all times, you will best be able to change your body composition by losing fat and adding lean muscle mass. Those subjects with the largest energy imbalances (those who were over 500 calories in either ingestion or expenditure) were the fattest, while those with the most balanced energy levels were the leanest. So if you eat only your three squares a day, you're creating terrific imbalances in your energy levels. Between meals, you're burning many more calories than you're taking in. At mealtimes, you're taking in many more than you're burning. Research shows that this kind of eating plan is great—if your dream is to be the next John Candy. But if you want to look slimmer, feel fitter, and—not coincidentally—live longer, then you need to eat more often. In the same study, subjects who added three snacks a day to three regular meals balanced out their energy better, lost fat, and increased lean body mass (as well as increased their power and endurance).

In a similar study, researchers in Japan found that boxers who ate the same amount of calories a day from either two or six meals both lost an average of 11 pounds in 2 weeks. But the guys who ate six meals a day lost 3 pounds more fat and 3 pounds less muscle than the ones who ate only two meals.

There's science to support the fact that more meals work, but the plain-speak reason it works is because it does something that many diets don't do: It keeps you full and satiated, which will reduce the likelihood of a diet-destroying binge.

How it works: For scheduling purposes, alternate your larger meals with smaller snacks. Eat two of your snacks roughly 2 hours before lunch and dinner, and one snack roughly 2 hours after dinner. Here's what it may look like:

> **8 a.m.: breakfast**
>
> **11 a.m.: snack**
>
> **1 p.m.: lunch**
>
> **4 p.m.: snack**
>
> **6 p.m.: dinner**
>
> **8 p.m.: snack**

For a complete 7-day meal plan, check out page 94. It's not something you need to stick to religiously, just a suggestion for how you can make the New Abs Diet work for you. It also shows how to incorporate the recipes you'll find in Chapter 9 into your everyday life.

Guideline 2: Make These 12 Abs Diet Powerfoods the Staples of Your Diet

THE NEW ABS DIET will teach you to focus on (not restrict yourself to) a handful of food types—the Abs Diet Power 12—to fulfill your core nutritional needs. These foods are all good for you. They're so good, in fact, that they'll just about single-handedly exchange your fat for muscle (provided you've kept your receipt). Just as important, I've designed the Power 12 to include literally thousands of food combinations. There are hundreds of dairy products, fruits and vegetables, lean meats, and other choices to satisfy your tastes. Incorporating these Abs Diet Powerfoods into your six meals a day will satiate your tastes and cravings and keep you from feasting on the dangerous fat promoters in your diet.

You'll read more about these powerfoods in Chapter 8. For now, I just want you to remember:

A lmonds and other nuts

B eans and legumes

S pinach and other green vegetables

D airy (fat-free or low-fat milk, yogurt, cheese)

I nstant oatmeal (unsweetened, unflavored)

E ggs

T urkey and other lean meats

P eanut butter

O live oil

W hole-grain breads and cereals

E xtra-protein (whey) powder

R aspberries and other berries

Guideline 3: Drink Smoothies Regularly

WITH SCHEDULES THE way they are today, it's no wonder that your definition of a kitchen gadget is the one with a team logo that can open bottles. You need to make one exception for the kitchen gadget that won't fit on a key chain: the blender. I don't care how many speeds it has or how it looks, and I couldn't tell you the difference between a mince and a frappe. All I care about is how much stuff I can put in it and how good the stuff tastes when it comes out. (One thing I do recommend: Get a blender with at least 400 watts, which will give it the power to handle chopping ice and shredding fruit and to outlast any Jimmy Buffett fans who might drop by unexpectedly.)

When you consider that changing your body takes time, motivation, and knowledge, consider your blender to be one of your most powerful tools in the

Abs Diet plan. Smoothies made with a mixture of the Abs Diet Powerfoods can act as meal substitutions and as potent snacks, and they work brilliantly for a few reasons.

▶ They require little time.

▶ Adding berries, flavored whey powder, or peanut butter will make them taste like dessert, which will satisfy your sweet cravings.

▶ Their thickness takes up a lot of space in your stomach.

I don't cook much. When I want a quick, healthy meal, I dump milk, low-fat vanilla yogurt, ice, uncooked instant oatmeal, peanut butter, and a couple of teaspoons of chocolate whey powder into my blender. You can mix and match ingredients, depending on your tastes (see the recipes in Chapter 9), but use the milk, yogurt, whey powder, and ice as the base. Here's the evidence showing these blended power drinks will help you control your weight:

▶ Researchers at Purdue University found that people stayed fuller longer when they drank thick drinks than when they drank thin ones—even when calories, temperatures, and amounts were equal.

▶ A Penn State study found that men who drank yogurt shakes that had been blended until they doubled in volume ate 96 fewer calories a day than men who drank shakes of normal thickness.

▶ In a study presented at the North American Association of the Study of Obesity, researchers found that regularly drinking meal replacements increased a man's chance of losing weight and keeping it off for longer than a year.

▶ A University of Tennessee study found that men who added three servings of yogurt a day to their diets lost 61 percent more body fat and 81 percent more stomach fat over 12 weeks than men who didn't eat yogurt. Wow! Researchers speculated that the calcium helps the body burn fat and limit the amount of new fat your body can make.

How it works: Drink an 8-ounce smoothie for breakfast, as a meal substitute, or as a snack before or after your workout.

Guideline 4: Stop Counting

THOUGH CALORIE BURNING is paramount to losing fat, calorie counting will make you lose focus and motivation. By eating these 12 Abs Diet Powerfoods and their many relatives, the foods themselves will, in a way, count your calories for you. They'll keep you healthy and feeling full and satisfied. Plus, the most energy-efficient foods are almost like doormen at a nightclub: They're not going to let any of the riffraff in without your approval.

Of course, that doesn't give you license to speed down the road of monstrous portions. Most of us claim that we watch what we eat, but most of us don't have a clue. A US Department of Agriculture study asked men what they ate, then checked it against reality. The truth: Men ages 25 to 50 were eating twice the grains, fats, and sweets that they estimated. If you eat six well-balanced meals, your body will regulate portions through things like fiber, protein, and the sheer volume of the smoothies. That said, it's always wise—especially in the beginning of the plan, when you're most vulnerable and adjusting to a new way of eating—to

‖‖‖

Obesity Risks

Almost as important as what you eat is when you eat. Researchers at the University of Massachusetts analyzed the eating habits of 500 women and men and found connections between the way people eat and the risk of becoming overweight.

HABIT	CHANGES YOUR RISK OF OBESITY BY
Eating at least one midday snack	–39 percent
Eating dinner as your biggest meal of the day	+6 percent
Waiting more than 3 hours after waking up to eat breakfast	+43 percent
Eating more than a third of your meals in restaurants	+69 percent
Going to bed hungry (3 or more hours after your last meal or snack)	+101 percent
Eating breakfast away from home	+137 percent
Not eating breakfast	+450 percent

focus on portion control by limiting the servings of some foods, especially the ones with fat (like peanut butter) and carbohydrates (like rice or bread). A good rule: Stick to one to two servings per food group, and keep the total contents of each meal contained to the diameter of your plate. A height restriction is in effect.

Guideline 5:
Know What to Drink—And What Not To

I DRINK BEER. I drink wine. I like to drink beer and wine, and gin and tonics on a hot summer day, and a lot of other things. There are health benefits to having one or two drinks a day, but there are many ways that alcohol can get you into trouble. Most important, alcohol—like soda—adds calories that you don't need right now. These calories are empty calories because they don't actually help make you full or decrease the amount of food you'll eat. In fact, alcohol makes you eat more and encourages your body to burn less fat. When Swiss researchers gave eight healthy men enough alcohol to exceed their daily calorie requirements by 25 percent (five beers for someone who eats 3,000 calories a day), they found that booze actually impaired men's ability to burn fat by as much as 36 percent. Booze also makes you store fat. Your body sees alcohol as a poison and tries to get rid of it. So your liver stops processing all other calories until it has dealt with the alcohol. Anything else you eat while you're drinking most likely will end up as fat. In some more indirect ways, alcohol can inhibit your body's production of testosterone and human growth hormone— two hormones that help burn fat and build muscle.

I hate to tell you to drink water, but drinking about eight glasses a day has a lot of benefits. It helps keep you satiated (a lot of times what we interpret as hunger is really thirst). Water flushes the waste products your body makes when it breaks down fat for energy or when it processes protein. You also need water to transport nutrients to your muscles, to help digest food, and to keep your metabolism clicking.

If you're serious about shedding belly flab, I'd encourage you to stay off the booze for the 6-week plan. At the least, limit yourself to two or three alcoholic drinks per week. The best drinks you can have are fat-free, 1 percent or 2 percent milk; water; and green tea (or, if you must, two glasses of diet soda a day).

(continued on page 96)

||||||||||||||||||||||||||||||||||||||||||||||||||||||||||||||||||||||||||||||||||||||||||||||||||||||

The 7-Day Abs Diet Meal Plan

Unlike most diet plans, which are laden with complex, hard-to-follow rules and verboten foods you love but have to live without, the New Abs Diet lets you eat the foods you love, keeps your cravings at bay, and helps you control stress—all at the same time. Here's an example of how you can structure a week of eating. It's not written in stone, by any means: Mix up the meals. Substitute whenever you want. Heck, I don't care if you eat the same thing every day for a week. The purpose of this chart is simply to show you how to follow the principles of the Abs Diet. So enjoy!

MONDAY

Breakfast: One tall glass (8 to 12 ounces) Abs Diet Ultimate Power Smoothie (page 129); make extra for later

Snack #1: 2 teaspoons peanut butter, raw vegetables (as much as you want)

Lunch: Turkey or roast beef sandwich on whole-grain bread, 1 cup 1 percent or fat-free milk, 1 apple

Snack #2: 1 ounce almonds, 1½ cups berries

Dinner: A Thinner Mexican Dinner (page 147)

Snack #3: 8 to 12 ounces Abs Diet Ultimate Power Smoothie

TUESDAY

Breakfast: Eggs Beneficial Sandwich (page 134)

Snack #1: 2 teaspoons peanut butter, 1 bowl oatmeal or high-fiber cereal

Lunch: The I-Am-Not-Eating-Salad Salad (page 140)

Snack #2: 3 slices deli turkey, 1 large orange

Dinner: Bodacious Brazilian Chicken (page 148)

Snack #3: 1 ounce almonds, 4 ounces cantaloupe

WEDNESDAY

Breakfast: One tall glass (8 to 12 ounces) Strawberry Field Marshall Smoothie (page 129); make extra for later

Snack #1: 1 ounce almonds, 1 ounce raisins

Lunch: The Johnny Apple Cheese Sandwich (page 139)

Snack #2: 1 stick string cheese, raw vegetables (as much as you want)

Dinner: Chile-Peppered Steak (page 148)

Snack #3: 8 to 12 ounces Strawberry Field Marshall Smoothie

II

THURSDAY

Breakfast: 1 slice whole-grain bread with 1 tablespoon peanut butter, 1 medium orange, 1 cup All-Bran cereal with 1 cup 1 percent or fat-free milk, 1 cup berries

Snack #1: 8 ounces low-fat yogurt, 1 can low-sodium V8 juice

Lunch: Guilt-Free BLT (page 141)

Snack #2: 3 slices deli roast beef, 1 large orange

Dinner: Philadelphia Fryers (page 149)

Snack #3: 2 teaspoons peanut butter, 1 cup low-fat ice cream

FRIDAY

Breakfast: One tall glass (8 to 12 ounces) Banana Split Smoothie (page 130)

Snack #1: 1 ounce almonds, 4 ounces cantaloupe

Lunch: Hot Tuna (page 142)

Snack #2: 3 slices deli roast beef, 1 large orange

Dinner: Chili Con Turkey (page 150)

Snack #3: 8 to 12 ounces Chocolate Pudding Milkshake (page 132)

SATURDAY

Breakfast: One tall glass (8 to 12 ounces) The Kitchen Sink Smoothie (page 128); make extra for later

Snack #1: 1 bowl high-fiber cereal, 1 cup low-fat yogurt

Lunch: Leftover Chili Con Turkey

Snack #2: 2 teaspoons peanut butter, 1 or 2 slices whole-grain bread

Dinner: Cheat meal! Have whatever you've been craving this week: beer and wings, beer and pizza, beer and bratwurst—anything you can dream of.

Snack #3: 8 to 12 ounces The Kitchen Sink Smoothie

SUNDAY

Breakfast: The I-Haven't-Had-My-Coffee-Yet Sandwich (page 136)

Snack #1: 2 teaspoons peanut butter, 1 can low-sodium V8 juice

Brunch (relax—it's Sunday): 2 scrambled eggs, 2 slices whole-grain toast, 1 banana, 1 cup 1 percent or fat-free milk

Snack #2: 3 slices deli roast beef, 1 slice fat-free cheese

Dinner: Tuna with Wasabi (page 149)

Snack #3: 1 ounce almonds, 1 cup low-fat ice cream

Guideline 6: For One Meal a Week, Forget the First Five Guidelines

I WOULD NEVER advocate cheating on your spouse, your employer, or your taxes. But I want you to cheat on this diet. I want you to take one meal during the week and forget everything about good carbohydrates and good fats. Have half a pizza, buffalo wings, or whatever it is that you miss the most while you're on this plan. Have it, savor it, and then dig back in for another week. I want you to cheat for a couple reasons. One, I want you to control when you cheat. Plan your cheat meal for the week—whether it's Saturday night out, during a football game, or whenever. But if you keep it planned, you'll stick to it. The way to control your cravings is to satisfy them every once in a while. If you can make it through 6 days, you reward yourself and know that 6 days of good eating is a regimen you can stick to over the long term. And there's another important reason I want you to cheat: because it'll actually help you change your body. A successful diet plan is about how you eat most of the time, not how you eat all of the time. In fact, a high-calorie day of eating can rev up your metabolism.

||||||||||||||||||||||||||||||||||||||||||||||||||||||||||||||||||||||||||||||||||||||||||||||||||||||||||||

Extra Credit

Turbocharge the six Abs Diet guidelines by establishing these three simple habits of lean and healthy eating.

1. Prepare your own meals. As your number of home-cooked meals increases, your fast-food visits decrease. By cooking at home using the recipes in the next chapter, you'll automatically avoid huge restaurant portions and calorie overload. USDA scientists found that people eat about 500 calories more a day when they consume food made outside the home.

2. Eliminate added sugars. "This is the simplest way to clean up any diet," says Jonny Bowden, PhD, The author of *The 150 Healthiest Foods on Earth.* Avoid putting sugar in anything you eat. And stay away from soda, baked goods, fruit drinks and sugary breakfast cereals. USDA researchers say 82 percent of our added sugar can be attributed to those foods.

3. Don't fear fat. Fats found in meat, dairy, avocados, olive oil, and nuts are filling and add flavor to meals, which will help you avoid feeling deprived, says nutritionist Alan Aragon, MS. For a rule of thumb, shoot for half a gram of fat for every pound of your desired body weight.

Researchers at the National Institutes of Health found that men who ate twice as many calories in a day as they normally did increased their metabolism by 9 percent in the 24-hour period that followed. But here's where you have to show control. I think that this diet plan allows you to have plenty of foods that are both good and good for you, but I know you will crave other foods that don't fit into our guidelines. Think of this cheat meal as the carrot at the end of a good week of eating. I encourage you to enjoy your meal of gluttony, and please, don't make the carrot literally a carrot.

Chapter 8

THE ABS DIET POWER 12

Meet the Powerfoods That Will Shrink Your Gut and Keep You Healthy for Life

I N THE PREVIOUS CHAPTER, I gave you the six guidelines for following the Abs Diet and touched briefly on the Abs Diet Power 12. Now, I want you to meet each of these 12 superheroes up close.

These 12 foods make up a large part of your diet. The more of these foods you eat, the better your body will be able to increase lean muscle mass and avoid storing fat. Though you can base entire meals and snacks around these foods, you don't have to. But do follow these guidelines.

▶ Incorporate two or three of these foods into each of your three major meals and at least one of them into each of your three snacks.

▶ Diversify your food at every meal to get a combination of protein, carbohydrates, and fat.

▶ Make sure you sneak a little bit of protein into each snack.

How to read the key: For at-a-glance scanning, I've included the following icons under the descriptions of each of the Abs Diet Powerfoods. Each icon
demonstrates which important roles each food can help play in maintaining
optimum health.

Builds muscle: Foods rich in muscle-building plant and animal proteins qualify for this seal of approval, as do foods rich in certain minerals linked to proper muscle maintenance, such as magnesium.

Helps promote weight loss: Foods high in calcium and fiber (both of
which protect against obesity) as well as foods that help build fat-busting muscle tissue earn this badge of respect.

Strengthens bone: Calcium and vitamin D are the most import-
ant bone builders, and they protect the body against osteoporosis.
But beware: High levels of sodium can leach calcium out of bone tissue.
Fortunately, all of the powerfoods are naturally low in sodium.

Lowers blood pressure: Any food that's not high in sodium can help
lower blood pressure—and score this designation—if it has beneficial
amounts of potassium, magnesium, or calcium.

Fights cancer: Research has shown that there is a lower risk of some
types of cancer among those people who maintain low-fat, high-fiber
diets. You can also help foil cancer by eating foods that are high in calcium,
beta-carotene, or vitamin C. In addition, all cruciferous (cabbage type) and
allium (onion type) vegetables get the cancer protection symbol because
research has shown they help prevent certain kinds of cancer.

Improves immune function: Vitamins A, E, B6, and C; folate; and the
mineral zinc help to increase the body's immunity to certain types of
disease. This icon indicates a powerfood with high levels of one or more of
these nutrients.

Fights heart disease: Artery-clogging cholesterol can lead to trouble
if you eat foods that are predominantly saturated and trans fats, while
foods that are high in monounsaturated or polyunsaturated fats will actually
help protect your heart by keeping your cholesterol levels in check.

#1: Almonds and Other Nuts

Superpowers: builds muscle, fights cravings

Secret weapons: protein, monounsaturated fats, vitamin E, fiber, magnesium, folate (peanuts), phosphorus

Fights against: obesity, heart disease, muscle loss, wrinkles, cancer, high blood pressure

Sidekicks: pumpkin seeds, sunflower seeds, avocados

Imposters: salted or smoked nuts

These days, you hear about good fats and bad fats the way you hear about good cops and bad cops. One's on your side, and one's gonna beat you silly. Oreos fall into the latter category, but nuts are clearly out to help you. They contain the monounsaturated fats that clear your arteries and help you feel full.

All nuts are high in protein and monounsaturated fat. But almonds are like Jack Nicholson in *One Flew over the Cuckoo's Nest*: They're the king of the nuts. A handful of almonds provides half the amount of vitamin E you need in a day and 8 percent of the calcium. They also contain 19 percent of your daily requirement of magnesium—a key component for muscle building. In a Western Washington University study, people taking extra magnesium were able to lift 20 percent more weight and build more muscle than those who weren't. A 2009 study in the *American Journal of Clinical Nutrition* showed that eating almonds suppresses hunger, and the more you chew them the greater your feelings of fullness will be. In the study, people who chewed 25 to 40 times absorbed more healthy monounsaturated fats and had higher levels of appetite-suppressing hormones than those who chewed just 10 times.

You can eat as much as two handfuls of almonds a day. A Toronto University study found that men can eat this amount daily without gaining any extra weight. A Purdue University study showed that people who ate nuts high in monounsaturated fat felt full an hour and a half longer than those who ate fat-free food (rice cakes, in this instance). If you eat 2 ounces of almonds (about 24 of them), it should be enough to suppress your appetite—especially if you wash them down with 8 ounces of water. The fluid helps expand the fiber in the nuts to help you feel fuller. Also, try to keep the nuts' nutrient-rich skins on them.

Here are ways to seamlessly introduce almonds into your diet:

▶ Add chopped almonds to plain peanut butter.

▶ Toss a handful on cereal, yogurt, or ice cream.

▶ Put slivers in an omelet.

▶ For a quick popcorn alternative: Spray a handful of almonds
with nonstick cooking spray, and bake at 400 degrees for 5 minutes.
Take them out of the oven, and sprinkle with either brown sugar
and cinnamon, or cayenne pepper and thyme.

But don't stop at almonds. Walnuts, pistachios, Brazil nuts, and pecans also deliver amazing health benefits. No food packs more selenium than Brazil nuts; 1 ounce has almost 10 times the recommended dietary allowance. University of Arizona scientists recently found that selenium may prevent colon cancer in men. Walnuts, on the other hand, are the only nuts that contain a significant amount of alpha-linolenic acid, the only type of omega-3 fat that you'll find in plant-based food. While chomping on walnuts, I want you to consider adding ground flaxseed to your food, which also provides omega-3s, plus 4 grams of fiber per tablespoon. Although not technically a nut, flaxseed has a nutty flavor, so you can add some to your meat or beans, spoon it over cereal, or add a tablespoon to a smoothie. One caveat,

‖‖

Eat Beans, Stay Lean

Studies show that regular bean eaters weigh less than those who don't eat beans. Check out some other superpowers of specific beans:

The antiaging agent: red kidney beans. This chili staple contains more antioxidants and omega-3s than any of its bean brethren, plus thiamine, which may be protective against Alzheimer's disease.

The heart healer: navy beans. They have the most cholesterol-clobbering fiber of any bean at 10.5 grams per 100-gram serving, plus tons of potassium.

The brain booster: black beans. Great in breakfast burritos, black beans are full of anthocyanins, compounds that have been shown to improve brain function.

before you get all nutty: Smoked and salted nuts don't make the cut here because of their high sodium content. High sodium can mean high blood pressure.

#2: Beans and Legumes

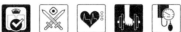

Superpowers: builds muscle, helps burn fat, regulates digestion

Secret weapons: fiber, protein, iron, folate

Fights against: obesity, colon cancer, heart disease, high blood pressure

Sidekicks: lentils, peas, bean dips, hummus, edamame

Imposters: refried beans, which are high in saturated fats; baked beans, which are high in sugar

Most of us can trace our resistance to beans to some unfortunately timed intestinal upheaval (third-grade math class, a first date gone awry). But beans are, as the song says, good for your heart; the more you eat them, the more you'll be able to control your hunger. Black, lima, pinto, garbanzo—you pick the bean (as long as it's not refried—refried beans are loaded with fat). Beans are a low-calorie food packed with protein, fiber, and iron—ingredients crucial for building muscle and losing weight. Gastrointestinal disadvantages notwithstanding, they serve as one of the key members of the Abs Diet cabinet

||||||||||||||||||||||||||||||||||||||||||||||||||||||||||||||||||||||||||||||||||||||||||||||||||

The muscle builder: soybeans. Technically a legume, soybeans are one of the only common plant foods that contain complete protein, making them terrific muscle-building meat substitues for vegetarians.

The cancer killer: lentils. Women who eat lentils frequently have a lower risk of developing breast cancer, says a study in the *International Journal of Cancer*. Other studies show that lentils may protect against prostate and colorectal cancers.

The diabetes destroyer: garbanzo beans. Also known as chickpeas, garbanzos are high in fiber, which helps stabilize blood sugar, lowering the risk of type 2 diabetes. Add them to salads and soups. Chickpeas (mashed) are the main ingredient in hummus, a garlicky bean spread that's terrific on crackers or as a healthier substitute for mayonnaise on sandwiches.

because of all their nutritional power. In fact, you can swap in a bean-heavy dish for a meat-heavy dish a couple of times per week; you'll be lopping a lot of saturated fat out of your diet and replacing it with higher amounts of fiber.

#3: Spinach and Other Green Vegetables

  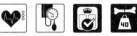

Superpowers: neutralizes free radicals, which are molecules that accelerate the aging process

Secret weapons: vitamins including A, C, and K; folate; minerals including calcium and magnesium; fiber; beta-carotene

Fights against: cancer, heart disease, stroke, obesity, osteoporosis

Sidekicks: cruciferous vegetables such as broccoli and brussels sprouts; and green, yellow, red, and orange vegetables such as asparagus, peppers, and yellow beans

Imposters: none, as long as you don't fry them or smother them in fatty cheeses

Lean Green Machines

Essentially, iceberg lettuce is the nutritional equivalent of a plastic office plant—it adds a little color, but mostly it just takes up space. Iceberg may be cheap and plentiful, but it contains almost no fiber, vitamins, or minerals. If you're going to eat salad, you might as well eat salad with some cojones to it. Check out this green dream team.

The cancer killer: romaine. This celery-flavored green is one of the best vegetable sources of beta-carotene—712 micrograms per cup. A University of Illinois study showed that high levels of beta-carotene inhibited the growth of prostate cancer cells by 50 percent.

The heart healer: endive. It's slightly bitter and a little crisp, and it offers twice the fiber of iceberg lettuce. A cup of endive also provides almost 20 percent of your daily requirement of folate. People who don't get enough of this essential B vitamin may have a 50 percent greater risk of developing heart disease.

The brain booster: mustard greens. These spicy, crunchy greens are packed with the amino acid tyrosine. In a recent US military study, researchers found

You know vegetables are packed with important nutrients, but they're also a critical part of your body-changing diet. I like spinach in particular because it's such an efficient vegetable: one serving supplies nearly a full day's worth of vitamin A and half of your vitamin C. It's also loaded with folate—a vitamin that protects against heart disease, stroke, and colon cancer. To incorporate it, you can take the fresh stuff and use it as lettuce on a sandwich, or try stir-frying it with a little fresh garlic and olive oil. You can always guarantee that you have spinach handy by stocking up on frozen spinach. Packed right after picking, the frozen stuff is full of the essential nutrients. And frozen spinach conveniently boosts the nutritional value of eggs, soups and sauces.

Another potent power vegetable is broccoli. It's high in fiber and more densely packed with vitamins and minerals than almost any other food. For instance, it contains nearly 90 percent of the vitamin C of fresh orange juice and almost half as much calcium as milk. It is also a powerful defender against diseases like cancer because it increases the enzymes that help detoxify carcinogens. Tip: With broccoli, you can skip the stalks. The florets have three times as much beta-carotene as the stems, and they're also a great source of other antioxidants.

||||||||||||||||||||||||||||||||||||||||||||||||||||||||||||||||||||||||||||||||||||||||||||||||||||||||||||||||||||

that eating a tyrosine-rich meal an hour before taking a test helped soldiers significantly improve both their memories and their concentration.

The bone builder: arugula. One cup has 10 percent of the bone-building mineral found in a glass of whole milk and 100 percent less saturated fat. There's also some magnesium in every bite, for more protection against osteoporosis.

The pipe protector: watercress. It's a pepper-flavored HEPA filter for your body. Watercress contains phytochemicals that may prevent cigarette smoke and other airborne pollutants from causing lung cancer.

The antiaging agent: bok choy. Think of it as a cabbage-flavored multivitamin. A bowl of bok choy has 23 percent of your daily requirement of vitamin A and a third of your vitamin C, along with three tongue-twisting, cancer-fighting, age-reducing phytochemicals: flavonoids, isothiocyanates, and dithiolthione.

The sight sharpener: spinach. Spinach is a top source of lutein and zeaxanthin, two powerful antioxidants that protect your vision from the ravages of old age. A Tufts University study found that frequent spinach eaters had a 43 percent lower risk of age-related macular degeneration.

If you hate vegetables, you can learn to hide them but still reap the benefits. Try pureeing them and adding them to marinara sauce or chili. The more you chop and puree vegetables, the more invisible they become and the easier it is for your body to absorb them. With broccoli, sauté it in garlic and olive oil, and douse it with hot sauce.

#4: Dairy (Fat-Free or Low-Fat Milk, Yogurt, Cheese, and Cottage Cheese)

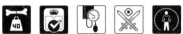

Superpowers: builds strong bones, fires up weight loss

Secret weapons: calcium, vitamins A and B12, riboflavin, phosphorus, potassium

Fights against: osteoporosis, obesity, high blood pressure, cancer

Sidekicks: none

Imposters: whole milk, frozen yogurt

Dairy is nutrition's version of a typecast actor. It gets so much attention for one thing it does well—strengthening bones—that it gets little or no attention for all the other stuff it does well. It's about time for dairy to accept a breakout role as a vehicle for weight loss. Just take a look at the mounting evidence: A University of Tennessee study found that dieters who consumed between 1,200 and 1,300 milligrams of calcium a day lost nearly twice as much weight as dieters getting less calcium. In a Purdue University study of 54 people, those who took in 1,000 milligrams of calcium a day (about 3 cups of fat-free milk) gained less weight over 2 years than those with low-calcium diets. Some researchers think that calcium probably prevents weight gain by increasing the breakdown of body fat and hampering its formation. Another theory, based on a new study in the *British Journal of Nutrition*, suggests that the brain may detect when the body isn't getting enough calcium and signal your body to eat more food to make up for the deficit. So, making sure you consume enough calcium can play an important role in your weight-loss efforts. Chow down on low-fat yogurt, cheeses, and other dairy products every day. But as your major source of calcium, I recommend milk for one primary reason: volume. Liquids can take up valuable room in your stomach and send the signal to your brain that you're full. Adding in a sprinkle of chocolate powder can also help curb sweet cravings while still providing nutritional power.

#5: Instant Oatmeal (Unsweetened, Unflavored)

Superpowers: boosts energy and sex drive, reduces cholesterol, maintains blood sugar levels

Secret weapons: complex carbohydrates and fiber

Fights against: heart disease, diabetes, colon cancer, obesity

Sidekicks: high-fiber cereals like All Bran and Fiber One

Imposters: cereals with added sugar and high-fructose corn syrup

Oatmeal is the Bo Derek of your pantry: It's a perfect 10. You can eat it at breakfast to propel you through sluggish mornings, a couple of hours before a workout to feel fully energized by the time you hit the weights, or at night to avoid a late-night binge. I recommend instant oatmeal for its convenience. But I want you to buy the unsweetened, unflavored variety and use other powerfoods such as milk and berries to enhance the taste. Preflavored oatmeal often comes loaded with sugar calories.

Oatmeal contains soluble fiber, meaning that it attracts fluid and stays in your stomach longer than insoluble fiber (like vegetables). Soluble fiber is thought to reduce blood cholesterol by binding with digestive acids made from cholesterol and sending them out of your body. When this happens, your liver has to pull cholesterol from your blood to make more digestive acids, and your bad cholesterol levels drop.

Trust me: You need more fiber, both soluble and insoluble. Doctors recommend we get between 25 and 35 grams of fiber per day, but most of us get half that. Fiber is like a bouncer for your body, kicking out troublemakers and showing them the door. It protects you from heart disease. It protects you from colon cancer by sweeping carcinogens out of the intestines quickly.

A Penn State study also showed that oatmeal sustains your blood sugar levels longer than many other foods, which keeps your insulin levels stable and ensures you won't be ravenous for the few hours that follow. That's good, because spikes in the production of insulin slow your metabolism and send a signal to the body that it's time to start storing fat. Since oatmeal breaks down slowly in the stomach, it causes less of a spike in insulin levels than foods like bagels. Include it in a smoothie or as your breakfast. (A US Navy study showed that simply eating breakfast raised metabolism by 10 percent.)

Another cool fact about oatmeal: Preliminary studies indicate that oatmeal raises the levels of free testosterone in your body, enhancing your body's ability to build muscle and burn fat and boosting your sex drive.

#6: Eggs

Superpowers: builds muscle, burns fat

Secret weapons: protein, vitamin B12, vitamin A

Fights against: obesity

Sidekicks: none

Imposters: none

For a long time, eggs were considered pure evil, and doctors were more likely to recommend tossing eggs at passing cars than into omelet pans. That's because just two eggs contain enough cholesterol to put you over your daily recommended value. Though you can cut out some of the cholesterol by removing part of the yolk and using the whites, more and more research shows that eating an egg or two a day will not raise your cholesterol levels, as once previously believed. In fact, we've learned that most blood cholesterol is made by the body from dietary fat, not dietary cholesterol. And that's why you should take advantage of eggs and their powerful makeup of protein.

Eggs have the highest "biological value" of protein—a measure of how well it supports your body's protein need—of any food. In other words, egg protein is more effective in building muscle than protein from other sources, even milk and beef. Eggs also contain vitamin B12, which is important for fat breakdown.

#7: Turkey and Other Lean Meats
(Lean Steak, Chicken, Fish)

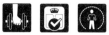

Superpower: builds muscle, improves the immune system

Secret weapons: protein, iron, zinc, creatine (beef), omega-3 fatty acids (fish), vitamins B6 (chicken and fish) and B12, phosphorus, potassium

Fights against: obesity, various diseases

Sidekicks: shellfish, Canadian bacon

Imposters: sausage, bacon, cured meats, ham, fatty cuts of steak like T-bone and rib-eye

A classic muscle-building nutrient, protein is the base of any solid diet plan. You already know that it takes more energy for your body to digest the protein in meat than it does to digest carbohydrates or fat, so the more protein you eat, the more calories you burn. Many studies support the notion that high-protein diets promote weight loss. In one study, researchers in Denmark found that men who substituted protein for 20 percent of their carbs were able to increase their metabolism and increase the number of calories they burned every day by up to 5 percent.

Among meats, turkey is a rare bird. Turkey breast is one of the leanest meats you'll find, and it packs nearly one-third of your daily requirements of niacin and vitamin B6. Dark meat, if you prefer, has lots of zinc and iron. Two cautions, though: If you're roasting a whole turkey for a family feast, avoid self-basting birds, which have been injected wth fat. And avoid eating the skin, which contains most of the fat.

Beef is another classic muscle-building protein. It's the top food source for creatine—the substance your body uses when you lift weights. Beef does have a downside: It contains saturated fats, but some cuts have more than others. Look for rounds or loins (that's code for extra-lean); sirloins and New York strips are less fatty than prime ribs and T-bones. And choose a smaller portion for your plate, which can help you lose weight without making you feel deprived. For example, by having a 6-ounce steak instead of an 8-ouncer, you'll save 140 calories, and still get 46 grams of muscle-building protein. Another tip: Wash down that steak with a glass of fat-free milk. Research shows that calcium (that magic bullet again!) may reduce the amount of saturated fat your body absorbs. Choose cuts on the left side of the chart. They contain less fat but still pack high amounts of protein.

LEAN BEEF (55 calories and 2 to 3 grams of fat per 1-ounce serving)	MEDIUM-FAT BEEF (75 calories and 5 grams of fat per 1-ounce serving)
Flank steak	Corned beef
Ground beef (extra-lean or lean)	Ground beef (not marked as lean or extra-lean)
London broil	Prime cut
Roast beef	
Tenderloin	

To cut down on saturated fats even more, concentrate on getting your protein from fish like tuna, salmon, and sardines, because they contain a healthy dose of omega-3 fatty acids. Omega-3s lower levels of a hormone called leptin in your body. Several recent studies suggest that leptin directly influences your metabolism: The higher your sustained leptin levels, the more readily your body stores calories as fat. Researchers at the University of Wisconsin found that mice with low leptin levels have faster metabolisms and are able to burn fat faster than animals with higher leptin levels. Mayo Clinic researchers studying the diets of two African tribes discovered that the tribe that ate fish frequently had leptin levels nearly five times lower than the tribe that primarily ate vegetables. A bonus benefit of learning how to fish: Researchers in Stockholm studied the diets of more than 6,000 men and found that those who ate no fish had three times the risk of prostate cancer than those who ate it regularly. It's the omega-3s that inhibit prostate cancer growth.

Whether you eat fish or not, consider taking omega-3 supplements. Also, I want you to consider adding ground flaxseed to your food. As I pointed out earlier, 1 tablespoon contains only 60 calories, but it packs in omega-3 fatty acids and has nearly 4 grams of fiber. It has a nutty flavor, so you can sprinkle it into a lot of different recipes, add some to your meat or beans, spoon it over cereal, or add a tablespoon to a smoothie.

III

Fat Content of Meat
(4 oz, raw, without skin or bone)

	TOTAL (G)	SATURATED (G)
Skinless chicken breast	1.41	0.37
Veal steak	2.45	0.74
Wild rabbit	2.63	0.78
Lean ground beef	4	1.50
Cured ham	4.68	1.56
Wild duck breast	4.82	1.50
Chicken drumstick	5.05	1.34
Lean pork tenderloin	5.06	1.79
Beef sirloin steak	5.15	2
Buffalo	5.44	2.31
Turkey leg	7.62	2.34
Turkey breast	7.96	2.17
Lean beef tenderloin	8.02	3
Lean pork chop	8.19	2.85
Porterhouse steak	8.58	3
Lean ground turkey	9.37	2.55
Veal breast meat	9.73	3.80
Rib-eye steak	18.03	7.30
T-bone steak	19.63	7.69
Ham	21.40	7.42
Pork belly	60.11	21.92
Cured pork	91.29	33.32

#8: Peanut Butter
(All-Natural, Sugar-Free)

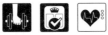

Superpowers: boosts testosterone, builds muscle, burns fat

Secret weapons: protein, monounsaturated fat, vitamin E, niacin, magnesium

Fights against: obesity, muscle loss, wrinkles, cardiovascular disease

Sidekicks: cashew and almond butters

Imposters: mass-produced sugary and trans fatty peanut butters

Yes, peanut butter has its disadvantages: It tends to stick to the roof of your mouth, it's high in calories, and it doesn't go over well when you order it in four-star restaurants. But it's packed with those heart-healthy monounsaturated fats that can increase your body's production of testosterone, which can help your muscles grow and your fat melt. In one 18-month experiment, people who integrated peanut butter into their diet maintained weight loss better than those on low-fat plans. A recent study from the University of Illinois showed that diners who had monounsaturated fats before a meal (in this case, it was olive oil) ate 25 percent fewer calories during that meal than those who didn't.

Practically speaking, peanut butter also works because it's a quick and versatile snack (keep a small jar handy at work to fend off hunger pangs). And it tastes great. Since a diet that includes an indulgence like peanut butter doesn't leave you feeling deprived, it's easier to follow and won't make you fall prey to craving for, say, glazed doughnuts or potato chips. Use PB on an apple, on the go, or to add flavor to potentially bland smoothies. For variety, try almond butter as a replacement for peanut butter on celery sticks or in a whole-wheat jelly sandwich. Nutrition-wise, almond butter offers a bit more fiber and vitamin E, and about the same amount of fat and calories. While we're on the topic of fat and calories, remember these two caveats: You shouldn't gorge on nut butters because of their high fat content; limit yourself to about 3 tablespoons per day. And you should stock up on all-natural peanut butter, not the mass-produced brands that have added sugar.

#9: Olive Oil

Superpowers: lowers cholesterol and boosts the immune system

Secret weapons: monounsaturated fat, vitamin E

Fights against: obesity, cancer, heart disease, high blood pressure

Sidekicks: canola oil, peanut oil, sesame oil

Imposters: vegetable and hydrogenated vegetable oils, trans fatty acids, margarine

You read extensive information on the value of high-quality fats like olive oil in Chapter 3. But it's worth reiterating here: Olive oil and its brethren will help you eat less by controlling your food cravings; they'll also help you burn fat and keep your cholesterol in check. Do you need any more reason to pass the bottle?

#10: Whole-Grain Breads and Cereals

Superpower: prevents your body from storing fat

Secret weapons: fiber, protein, thiamin, riboflavin, niacin, pyridoxine, vitamin E, magnesium, zinc, potassium, iron, calcium

Fights against: obesity, cancer, high blood pressure, heart disease

Sidekicks: brown rice, whole-wheat pretzels, whole-wheat pastas

Imposters: processed bakery products like white bread, bagels, and doughnuts; breads labeled wheat instead of whole wheat

There's only so long a person can survive on an all-protein diet or an all-salad diet or an all-anything diet. You will crave carbohydrates because your body needs carbohydrates. The key is to eat the ones that have been the least processed—carbs that still have all their heart-healthy, belly-busting fiber intact.

Grains such as wheat, corn, oats, barley, and rye are seeds that come from grasses, and they're broken into three parts—the germ, the bran, and the endosperm. Think of a kernel of corn. The biggest part of the kernel—the part that blows up when you make popcorn—is the endosperm. Nutritionally it's pretty much a big dud. It contains starch, a little protein, and some B vitamins. The germ is the smallest part of the grain; in the corn kernel, it's that little white seedlike thing. But while it's small, it packs the most nutritional power. It contains protein, oils, and the B vitamins thiamin, riboflavin, niacin, and pyridoxine. It also has vitamin E and the minerals magnesium, zinc, potassium, and iron. The bran is the third part of the grain and the part where all the fiber is stored. It's a coating around the endosperm that contains B vitamins, zinc, calcium, potassium, magnesium, and other minerals.

So what's the point of this little biology lesson? Well, get this: When food manufacturers process and refine grains, guess which two parts get tossed out? Yup, the bran, where all the fiber and minerals are, and the germ, where all the protein and vitamins are. And what they keep—the nutritionally bankrupt endosperm (that is, starch)—gets made into pasta, bagels, white bread, white rice, and just about every other wheat product and baked good you'll find. Crazy, right? But if you eat products made with all the parts of the grain—whole-grain bread, pasta, long-grain rice—you get all the nutrition that food manufacturers are otherwise trying to cheat you out of.

Whole-grain carbohydrates can play an important role in a healthy lifestyle. In an 11-year study of 16,000 middle-age people, researchers at the University of Minnesota found that consuming three daily servings of whole grains can reduce a person's mortality risk over the course of a decade by 23 percent. (Tell that to your buddy who's eating low-carb.) Whole-grain bread keeps insulin levels low, which keeps you from storing fat. In this diet, it's especially versatile because it'll supplement any kind of meal with little prep time. Toast for breakfast, sandwiches for lunch, with a dab of peanut butter for a snack. Don't believe the hype. Carbs—the right kind of carbs—are good for you.

Warning: Food manufacturers are very sneaky. Sometimes, after refining away all the vitamins, fiber, and minerals from wheat, they'll add molasses to the bread, turning it brown, and put it on the grocery shelf with a label that says wheat bread. It's a trick! Truly nutritious breads and other products will say whole wheat or whole grain. Don't be fooled.

#11: Extra-Protein (Whey) Powder

Superpowers: builds muscle, burns fat

Secret weapons: protein, cysteine, glutathione

Fights against: obesity

Sidekick: ricotta cheese

Imposter: soy protein

Protein powder? What the heck is that? It's the only Abs Diet Power-food that you may not be able to find at the supermarket, but it's the one that's worth the trip to a health food store. I'm talking about powdered whey protein, a type of animal protein that packs a muscle-building wallop. If you add whey powder to your meal—in a smoothie, for instance—you may very well have created the most powerful fat-burning meal possible. Whey protein is a high-quality protein that contains essential amino acids that build muscle and burn fat. But it's especially effective because it has the highest amount of protein for the fewest number of calories, making it fat's kryptonite. Smoothies with some whey powder can be most effective before a workout. A 2001 study at the University of Texas found that lifters who drank a shake containing amino acids and carbohydrates before working out increased their protein synthesis (their ability to build muscle) more than lifters who drank the same shake after exercising. Because exercise increases blood flow to tissues, the theory goes that having whey protein in your system when you work out may lead to a greater uptake of amino acids—the building blocks of muscle—in your muscle.

But that's not all. Whey protein can help protect your body from prostate cancer. Whey is a good source of cysteine, which your body uses to build a prostate cancer–fighting antioxidant called glutathione. Adding just a small amount may increase glutathione levels in your body by up to 60 percent.

By the way, the one great source of whey protein in your supermarket is ricotta cheese. Unlike other cheeses, which are made from milk curd, ricotta is made from whey, the liquid drained off during the making of cheeses like mozzarella. It's yet another good reason to visit your local Italian eatery.

#12: Raspberries and Other Berries

Superpowers: protects your heart; enhances eyesight; improves balance, coordination, and short-term memory; prevents cravings

Secret weapons: antioxidants, fiber, vitamin C, tannins (cranberries)

Fights against: heart disease, cancer, obesity

Sidekicks: most other fruits, especially apples and grapefruit

Imposters: jellies, most of which eliminate fiber and add sugar

Depending on your taste, any berry will do (except Crunch Berries). I like raspberries as much for their power as for their taste. They carry powerful levels of antioxidants, all-purpose compounds that help your body fight heart disease and cancer; the berry's flavonoids may also help your eyesight, balance, coordination, and short-term memory. One cup of raspberries packs 6 grams of fiber and more than half of your daily requirement of vitamin C.

Blueberries are also loaded with the soluble fiber that, like oatmeal, keeps you fuller longer. In fact, they're one of the most healthful foods you can eat. Blueberries beat out 39 other fruits and vegetables in the antioxidant power ratings. (One study also found that rats that ate blueberries were more coordinated and smarter than rats that didn't.) Psst: Frozen blueberries are just as good for you as the fresh ones.

Strawberries contain another valuable form of fiber called pectin (as do grapefruits, peaches, and oranges). In a study from the *Journal of the American College of Nutrition*, subjects drank plain orange juice or juice spiked with pectin. The people who got the loaded juice felt fuller after drinking it than those who got the juice without the pectin. The difference lasted for an impressive 4 hours.

Apples, known as "nature's toothbrush," are also rich in pectin fiber. A recent Penn State study demonstrated the fiber's power as a weight-loss tool: People who ate an apple 15 minutes before lunch ended up consuming 187 fewer calories during the meal than those who didn't snack beforehand. And all that apple chomping isn't just a good workout for your jaw; it tricks your brain into thinking you're eating more than you really are, say the researchers.

THE ABS DIET POWER 12

||||||||||||||||||||||||||||||||||||||||||||||||||||||||||||||||||||||||||||||||||||||||||||||||||||||

How to Pick Produce

A lot of us grew up with an aversion to fruits and vegetables, sometimes caused by doting moms who boiled canned greens into pulp and then insisted that by not eating them, we were somehow responsible for kids in China not having enough rice. Today, you've got two ways to prove your mom wrong: first, by showing her how really delicious fresh produce can be, if you know how to pick it and prepare it; and second, by showing her a picture of Yao Ming. (Hey, somebody was getting enough rice.)

Avocados. Feel for firm flesh. Toss back avocados with sunken, mushy spots. They should not rattle when shaken; that's a sign the pit has pulled away from the flesh.

Berries. Before you buy raspberries or strawberries, flip the carton over. You're looking for nature's expiration date: juice stains. You want berries you can eat without looking like you've been fingerprinted.

Cantaloupe. Don't knock on a melon to check its ripeness; slap it instead. You're listening for a hollow ring, not a dull thud or an inhuman scream.

Corn on the cob. The sweetest ears are slightly immature, with kernels that don't go all the way to the end of the cob. Toss 'em, husks and all, onto a medium-hot grill. Cook for 10 minutes, then peel back all but the last layer of husk. Grill 5 more minutes for that just-smoked flavor.

Kale. The smaller the leaves, the more tender the kale. Avoid wilted foliage with discolored spots. You want moist leaves with a dark blue-green color.

Peaches. Look for well-colored fruit with no green spots. The flesh should yield slightly when lightly pressed and should have a fragrant aroma. (Fragrant like a peach, not fragrant like your cousin Freddy.)

Tomatoes. Look for tomatoes that are firm and heavy for their size. They should have a sweet tomato aroma. If you generally don't like tomatoes, try the yellow kind; they tend to have a sweeter, less acidic flavor than red varieties.

Watermelon. Forget color, shape, or size: Watermelons are best judged by weight. The heavier a melon is, the more water it contains, and water is what helps give a melon its flavor.

Special Report

YOUR WEIGHT IS NOT YOUR FAULT

The Sneaky Ways Food Manufacturers Are Scheming to Make You Fat

T HE SEVEN NUTRITIONAL guidelines of the New Abs Diet and the Abs Diet Power 12 will steer you down the street of good eating. Follow those principles, and you will soon see remarkable changes in your appearance and your health. Now, I can take you down the street and show you the roads that lead you to a life of more muscle and less fat, but I'd be one shoddy tour guide if I didn't warn you of the two biggest hoodlums lurking around the corner. They're the two ingredients that will sneak up on you and rob you of all of the progress you've made on the diet: high-fructose corn syrup (HFCS) and trans fat. Luckily, thanks to the work of some scientific sketch artists, we have a pretty good idea of how they operate and when they strike.

And they strike often. These two new calorie bombs were hardly ever eaten before the mid-1970s, but now they're lurking in all sorts of foods. No wonder a recent study by the Centers for Disease Control and Prevention found that in 1971, American men averaged a daily intake of 2,450 calories and that women ate an average of 1,542, but in the year 2000, American men were averaging about 2,618 calories (up 7 percent), while women were eating 1,877 calories (up 22 percent). Did we all get hungrier? No. Our food got supersized—and so did we.

Now remember: This diet isn't about restriction or deprivation, so I'm not going to tell you to turn away and run every time you see HFCS or trans fats. What I do want you to do is get to know them. Know what foods they come in, and understand how they can destroy all the good things you've done to change your body. See, one of the secrets to the success of the Abs Diet is that it incorporates ways to deal with this terrible twosome. By eating six balanced

Substitute Teaching

Partially hydrogenated oils are everywhere. You can't eliminate them from your diet, but if you pick the right brands of the foods you love, you can dramatically reduce the amount you're taking in on a daily basis.

IF YOU WANT	PICK THIS TRANS FAT-FREE OPTION
Candy bar	Dove dark chocolate bar
Cereal	Kellogg's Frosted Mini Wheats or Post Premium Raisin Bran
Cheese spread	Cheez Whiz Light
Cookies	Archway fat-free cookies or Pamela's Gourmet cookies
Corn chips	Tostitos Natural yellow corn chips
Crackers	Wheatables original reduced-fat crackers
Fish sticks	Van de Kamp's Crisp & Healthy breaded fish sticks
French fries	McCain Shoestring 5-Minute French-Fried Potatoes
Frozen waffles	Kellogg's Special K fat-free waffles
Margarine	I Can't Believe It's Not Butter Fat-Free Spread or Smart Balance Light Spread
Popcorn	Air-popped popcorn
Potato chips	Ruffles Natural sea-salted, reduced-fat chips
Pot pies	Amy's organic pot pies
Stuffing	Butterball One-Step seasoned stuffing

meals and snacks with ingredients that increase your metabolism, you'll have less of a craving for foods that contain the bad substances. And by allowing yourself one cheat meal per week, you can schedule a place where you indulge in some of your favorite foods that fall into the criminal category. Instead of resisting them all the time, give them an occasional wave, but know that it's in your best interest not to make too many trips to this side of town.

High-Fructose Corn Syrup

PLAY WORD ASSOCIATION with high-fructose corn syrup, and if you're like me, you say, "Froot Loops." But when nutritionists play the same game, they spit out another word: obesity. HFCS is a man-made sweetener that's cheaper and sweeter than sugar. Food manufacturers love it because it enhances their profits, so they add it into an unbelievable number of foods. Cereal. Ketchup. Soda. Pasta sauce. Cookies. Even some meal replacement bars, which are supposed to be good for you, list HFCS way up high on the ingredients list.

We're talking about a processed sweetener that didn't even exist in the food chain until the 1970s. And HFCS is really, really, really bad for you. That's because it's packed with calories, but your body doesn't recognize these calories. In fact, HFCS shuts off your body's natural appetite control switches, so you can eat and eat and eat far beyond what your body would normally be able to handle. You probably know guys who can down a 2-liter bottle of Coke in a single sitting. Well, guess what? Before HFCS was invented, humans couldn't do that. Our natural appetite control switches would kick in, detect the sugar we were consuming, and say "¡No más!" But by shutting off the switches that control appetite, HFCS—a true junk food—is making America fat. In 1970, Americans ate about half a pound of HFCS per person per year. By the late 1990s, every person was consuming about 62 pounds every year. That's 228 additional calories per person per day.

The problem with HFCS is not the corn syrup; it's the fructose—a sugar that occurs naturally in fruit and honey. Corn syrup is primarily made of glucose, which can be burned as a source of immediate energy, stored in your liver or muscles for later use, or, as a last resort, turned to fat. But corn syrup isn't as sweet as other sugars, which is why HFCS became so popular. It's cheap and doubly sweet.

Unlike glucose, your body doesn't use fructose as an immediate source of energy; it metabolizes it into fat. While the small amount of fructose you get naturally through fruit and honey won't make you fat, eating HFCS is sort of like setting up an IV that pumps fat directly to your gut. One of the worst offenders is soft drinks: Soda consumption has doubled from 25 to 50 gallons per person per year in the last few decades. So the amount of HFCS we're getting is unprecedented—and many researchers think there's a direct link between the huge amount of HFCS we're consuming and the huge numbers we're seeing on the scale.

Go back to what you know about carbohydrates. When you eat any carbohydrate—whether it contains glucose or starch—your body releases insulin to regulate your body weight. First, it tries to push the carbs into your muscle cells to be used as energy and facilitates carb storage in the liver for later use. Then it suppresses your appetite, telling your body that you've had enough. Finally, it stimulates production of another protein, leptin, which is manufactured in your fat cells. In essence, leptin helps regulate how much fat you store and helps increase your metabolism to keep your weight in check. Like the mother-in-law who tries to tell you how to raise your kids, fructose screws up a system that was working perfectly fine without it. Fructose doesn't stimulate insulin and therefore doesn't increase the production of leptin—and that's the most important argument against fructose and HFCS: Without insulin and leptin, your body has no shut-off mechanism. You can drink 4 liters of Coke or down half a gallon of frozen yogurt, and your body thinks you haven't eaten since the last time Bill Gates borrowed money from his dad.

Soft drinks are one of the main sources of HFCS, but researchers tried to determine whether soda itself or HFCS was the problem. The verdict: HFCS. In a study in the *American Journal of Clinical Nutrition*, researchers took two groups of overweight people and had one group drink regular soft drinks while the other group drank diet soda (which contains no HFCS) for 10 weeks. The regular soda group gained weight and increased their body fat, as well as saw an increase in their blood pressure. The diet soda group consumed fewer calories than they normally would, lost weight, reduced body fat, and lowered blood pressure.

Even if you aren't a soda drinker, HFCS can still sneak up on you. Here's where nutritional labels come in handy. If a label says "sugar" or "cane sugar," the product contains sucrose, which is a 50/50 blend of glucose and fructose. That doesn't seem to be much of a problem. If HFCS is listed first or second, look at the chart on the nutrition label to see how much sugar the food contains. If it's just a gram or two, don't sweat it. But if you see a food that has 8 or more grams of sugar and HFCS is prominent on the list of ingredients, do what you do when you get turned down for a date: Move along to something else. The body can deal with a little of anything, but when your HFCS numbers start looking like Michael Jordan's career statistics, that's when you're headed for trouble. Consult the substitution chart for low-maintenance fixes.

FOODS HIGH IN HFCS OR FRUCTOSE	REPLACE WITH
Regular soft drinks	Unsweetened sparkling water or diet soda
Commercial candy (like jelly beans)	Chocolate candy (check the label; some chocolate bars have HFCS)
Pancake syrup	Real maple syrup
Frozen yogurt	Ice cream
Fruit-flavored yogurt	Organic yogurt
Highly sweetened cereals	Sugar-free or low-sugar cereals
Pasta sauce	Sugar-free pasta sauce
Energy bars	HFCS-free energy bars

Trans Fats

I TOUCHED ON trans fats in Chapter 4, but they're so bad for you that I want to revisit them here. Used in thousands of common prepared foods, from frozen waffles to Oreo cookies, french fries to bran muffins, trans fats are simply vegetable oil infused with hydrogen. You may not have heard much about it, because until 2003, companies weren't required to list trans fats on their nutritional labels.

Trans fats are difficult to digest, so they increase the amount of bad cholesterol in your blood and can dramatically boost your risk of heart disease, weaken your immune system, and even cause diabetes. Scientists have estimated that trans fats contribute to more than 30,000 premature deaths every year.

In the 1950s, scientists first made the link between saturated fat, cholesterol, and heart disease. After the discovery, manufacturers scrambled to find a way to cut saturated fats. Their solution was a process called partial hydrogenation, in which vegetable oil is combined with hydrogen and heated to extremely high temperatures. As the molecules in the oil warm up, they bond with the hydrogen, transforming a liquid to a solid. Voilà, trans fatty acid. Immediately, it was a hit. Restaurants liked it because they could fill their fry vats with it and keep it hot without smoking up their kitchens. Trans fatty acid was cheaper than butter and lasted longer, so restaurants could buy it in bulk without worrying about it spoiling. It soon became the staple of what you find in those two or three sinful supermarket aisles—chips and cookies. Trans fat made potato chips crispier and gave manufacturers a way to add the great taste of fat in ways it never had before—like Oreo cookie filling.

Since trans fat doesn't exist in nature, your body has a much harder time processing it than it does other types of fats. If your body were a subway system, the first stop trans fat would make would be at your heart. Trans fat increases your bad cholesterol and lowers your good cholesterol, and it increases blood levels of a compound called lipoprotein. The more lipoprotein you have in your system, the greater your risk of developing heart disease. Researchers have even found that trans fat could increase your risk of cancer.

After years of struggling with the food industry (which didn't want to list trans fat, for fear that consumers' knowing about it would result in the losses of millions or billions of dollars every year), the US Food and Drug Administration passed a regulation in mid-2003 that forces companies to list trans fat on food labels. But companies are free to phase in the change, meaning you won't see trans fat listed on all ingredient labels for years. In the meantime, here are some things you can do to limit the amount of trans fat in your diet.

AT THE GROCERY STORE	AT HOME	AT A RESTAURANT
Check the ingredients list for hydrogenated or partially hydrogenated. The higher these ingredients are on the label, the more trans fats the product contains (with the exception of peanut butter, which contains trace amounts).	Pick high-protein breakfasts like eggs or Canadian bacon instead of waffles. If you have toast, use peanut butter instead of margarine.	Ask what kind of oil the chef uses. You want to hear olive oil—not shortening.

AT THE GROCERY STORE	AT HOME	AT A RESTAURANT
Decode the food label. Add all the fat grams together that are listed on the label, and then subtract that number from the total fat content. The number you're left with is the estimate for the amount of trans fat in the food.	Snack on baked chips or chips fried in olive oil instead of ones with vegetable shortening (check the ingredients list).	Order foods that are baked, broiled, or grilled—not fried.
Buy margarine that is free of trans fat, like Smart Balance Light. Squeezable margarine also has less trans fat than the stick kind.	Flavor vegetables or baked potatoes with olive oil, sesame oil, or even butter-flavored spray instead of margarine.	Avoid bread, which may be filled with trans fat. It's better to pick a baked potato, soup, or salad.
Translate the labels. Cholesterol-free doesn't mean it's free of trans fat. Only fat-free means that.	Make a sandwich with a tortilla wrap or a pita instead of bread.	Blot oil from your fries as quickly as possible. A napkin can absorb excess grease.

Partially hydrogenated oils are in thousands of foods. You can't eliminate them entirely, but the National Institute of Medicine recommends cutting as many grams of trans fat as you can from your diet. Here's how some popular foods stack up.

FOOD		TRANS FAT (G)
1	chicken pot pie	8
2	biscuits	8
1	large order of fries	7
1	order of nachos with cheese	5
1	tablespoon of stick margarine	5
6	Oreos	4
1	waffle	4
1	small movie theater popcorn	3.5
1	slice of apple pie	3

Chapter 9

THE NEW ABS DIET MEAL PLAN
Using Powerfoods in Quick and Easy Recipes

IF YOU'RE LIKE A LOT OF people I know, you spend more time in the bathroom than you do in the kitchen. You simply don't have time to cook. You grab breakfast on your way out, fill up on coffee when you get there, eat lunch with coworkers or clients, and swing by the vending machine at 4. By the time you get home at 8, 9, or 10 o'clock, there are only two things you feel like doing—and both of them happen in your bed.

Look, I'm exactly the same way. I don't have the time, energy, or creative impulse to cook. My stovetop is more likely to be littered with bills and junk mail than pots and pans, and my oven is more likely to be used for storage than for cooking. (Once, my mom came for a visit and accidentally baked my basketball.) The first time I cooked dinner for a girlfriend, she accurately identified the meal as "some kind of meat."

So what you're going to see on the next few pages has been extensively idiot-proofed, and if you can operate a blender, a can opener, and a frying pan, you can handle these meals.

Most of these recipes are ones you can make quickly—some in less than 5 minutes. I also know that you're not going to make every meal, so I've included sample combinations of foods that make properly balanced meals, utilizing the powerfoods. For the dinners, servings sizes are larger than one, so you can also use the leftovers for lunch.

Abs Diet Smoothies

SMOOTHIES ARE ONE of the best parts about being on the New Abs Diet. They take less than 3 minutes to make. They pack in multiple high-nutrient foods. They fill you up. If that's not enough, they can also taste like a five-star dessert. You can come up with your own concoctions by using 1 percent milk, low-fat vanilla yogurt, whey powder, and ice as the main ingredients. Oatmeal and fruit make nice additions, as does a spoonful of peanut butter. Include all ingredients in a blender, and blend until smooth. For extra volume, add more ice. Here are some examples.

▶ FROM THE NEW ABS DIET COOKBOOK!

The Kitchen Sink (number of powerfoods: 6)

1   cup low-fat plain yogurt

1   cup ice cubes

¾   cup Fiber One cereal

1   scoop vanilla whey protein

1   teaspoons ground flaxseed

1   cup frozen strawberries or blueberries

1   handful fresh baby spinach

Makes: 1½ servings

Per serving: 310 calories, 21 g protein, 29 g carbohydrates, 10 g fat (4 g saturated fat), 220 mg sodium, 19 g fiber

Abs Diet Ultimate Power Smoothie (number of powerfoods: 5)

1 cup 1 percent milk

2 tablespoons low-fat vanilla yogurt

¾ cup instant oatmeal, nuked in water

2 teaspoons peanut butter

2 teaspoons chocolate whey powder

6 ice cubes, crushed

Makes: 2 8-ounce servings

Per serving: 220 calories, 12 g protein, 29 g carbohydrates, 4 g fat (1.5 g saturated fat), 118 mg sodium, 3 g fiber

Strawberry Field Marshall Smoothie (number of powerfoods: 5)

½ cup low-fat vanilla yogurt

1 cup 1 percent milk

2 teaspoons peanut butter

1 cup frozen strawberries

2 teaspoons whey powder

6 ice cubes, crushed

Makes: 2 8-ounce servings

Per serving: 186 calories, 11 g protein, 26 g carbohydrates, 5 g fat (2 g saturated fat), 151 mg sodium, 3 g fiber

Cereal Killer (number of powerfoods: 4)

½ cup All-Bran Extra Fiber cereal

1 cup 1 percent milk

½ cup blueberries

1 tablespoon honey

2 teaspoons whey powder

6 ice cubes, crushed

Makes: 2 8-ounce servings

Per serving: 145 calories, 8 g protein, 32 g carbohydrates, 2 g fat (1 g saturated fat), 155 mg sodium, 9 g fiber

Banana Split Smoothie (number of powerfoods: 3)

1 banana

½ cup low-fat vanilla yogurt

⅛ cup frozen orange juice
  concentrate

½ cup 1 percent milk

2 teaspoons whey powder

6 ice cubes, crushed

Makes: 2 8-ounce servings

Per serving: 171 calories, 8 g protein, 33 g carbohydrates, 2 g fat
(1 g saturated fat), 94 mg sodium, 2 g fiber

Halle Berries Smoothie (number of powerfoods: 4)

¾ cup instant oatmeal,
  nuked in water or fat-free milk

¾ cup fat-free milk

¾ cup mixed frozen blueberries,
  strawberries, and raspberries

2 teaspoons whey powder

3 ice cubes, crushed

Makes: 2 8-ounce servings

Per serving: 144 calories, 7 g protein, 27 g carbohydrates, 1 g fat
(0 g saturated fat), 109 mg sodium, 4 g fiber

PB&J Smoothie (number of powerfoods: 5)

¾ cup low-fat vanilla yogurt

¾ cup 1 percent milk

2 teaspoons peanut butter

1 medium banana

½ cup frozen unsweetened
  strawberries

2 teaspoons whey powder

4 ice cubes, crushed

Makes: 2 8-ounce servings

Per serving: 235 calories, 11 g protein, 39 g carbohydrates, 5 g fat
(2 g saturated fat), 154 mg sodium, 4 g fiber

Belly-Busting Berry (number of powerfoods: 6)

1 scoop low-fat vanilla ice cream

¼ cup each frozen blueberries, strawberries, and raspberries

½ cup low-fat milk

1 tablespoon vanilla whey protein powder

3 ice cubes

Makes: 1 8-ounce serving

Per serving: 251 calories, 15 g protein, 38 g carbohydrates, 4 g fat (2 g saturated fat), 116 mg sodium, 4 g fiber

Summer Smoothie (number of powerfoods: 4)

⅔ cup frozen strawberries

1 banana

½ cup cubed honeydew melon

4 ounces low-fat vanilla yogurt

¾ cup 1 percent milk

2 teaspoons vanilla whey powder

3 ice cubes, crushed

Makes: 2 8-ounce servings

Per serving: 199 calories, 9 g protein, 39 g carbohydrates, 2 g fat (1 g saturated fat), 117 mg sodium, 4 g fiber

||||||||||||||||||||||||||||||||||||||||||||||||||||||||||||||||||||||||||||||||||||||||||||||||

How to Pick a Better Yogurt

Shoot for more protein: Greek yogurt contains up to 18 grams of protein per serving (three times the amount in some regular yogurts).

Hunt for calcium: Choose a yogurt that contains at least 20 percent of your daily calcium needs. Men and women should get at least 1,000 mg a day; 1,200 mg after age 50.

Keep the calorie count around 100: Plain yogurt contains a relatively small amount of natural sugar and hovers around 100 calories. The sweeter flavored fruit yogurts can contain 170 calories per serving.

Make it better: If you want a sweeter yogurt, add a healthy sugar, such as blueberries or raisins. Toss in some walnuts or almonds for added nutrition.

Show Me the Honey (number of powerfoods: 3)

1 scoop low-fat butter pecan ice cream	1 teaspoon ground flaxseed
½ cup low-fat milk	1 dash cinnamon
1 tablespoon vanilla whey protein powder	1 teaspoon honey
	3 ice cubes

Makes: *1 8-ounce serving*

Per serving: *250 calories, 15 g protein, 38 g carbohydrates, 4 g fat (2 g saturated fat), 131 mg sodium, 3 g fiber*

▶ **FROM THE NEW ABS DIET COOKBOOK!**

Chocolate Pudding Milk Shake (number of powerfoods: 1)

3 cups cold fat-free milk	1 package (4 servings) Jell-O instant sugar-free chocolate pudding mix
1½ cups vanilla ice cream	

Makes: *5 servings*

Per serving: *190 calories, 8 g protein, 31 g carbohydrates, 4.5 g fat (3 g saturated fat), 650 mg sodium, 2 g fiber*

Abs Diet Breakfasts

BETWEEN GETTING A shower, skimming the paper, and the last-minute gluing you need to do on Bub's science fair project, breakfast is the martyr meal of the day. You usually sacrifice it for anything else that needs your attention. But if you had to rank the six meals in order of importance, the first meal would rank first. Breakfast wakes up your metabolism and tells it to start burning fat, decreasing your risk of obesity. The quickest way to incorporate the New Abs Diet into your breakfast is to combine potent foods (specifically the 12 Abs Diet Powerfoods) to make meals, such as:

▶ 8-ounce smoothie

▶ 2 tablespoons of peanut butter on whole-grain toast and 2 slices of Canadian bacon

▶ 1¾ cups of Shredded Wheat and Bran with 1 cup of 1 percent milk, 3 links of turkey sausage, and ½ cup of berries

▶ 2 scrambled eggs, 2 slices of whole-grain toast, 1 banana, and 1 cup of 1 percent or fat-free milk

▶ Cereal made with ¾ cup of high-fiber cereal, ¼ cup of Cap'n Crunch, 2 tablespoons of almonds, and 3/4 cup of 1 percent or fat-free milk

▶ 1 slice of whole-grain bread with 1 tablespoon of peanut butter, 1 medium orange, ½ cup of All-Bran cereal with ½ cup of 1 percent or fat-free milk, and ½ cup berries

On the weekends or on mornings when you can spare a few more minutes, these breakfasts will also deliver the appropriate nutritional punch.

▶ FROM THE NEW ABS DIET COOKBOOK!

Overtime Oats (number of powerfoods: 3)

4½ cups water	**½** teaspoon salt
1 cup steel-cut oats	**18** walnut halves
½ cup oat bran	**2** large strawberries, sliced

Mix the water, oats, oat bran, and salt in a medium saucepan. Bring to a boil over medium-high heat. Reduce the heat and cover the pan. Simmer, stirring frequently, for 30 minutes or until thickened. Serve topped with the walnuts and strawberries.

Makes: 3 1-cup servings

Per serving: 220 calories, 8 g protein, 31 g carbohydrates, 11 g fat (1.5 g saturated fat), 400 mg sodium, 6 g fiber

Eggs Beneficial Sandwich (number of powerfoods: 5)

1 large whole egg	1 slice Canadian bacon
3 large egg whites	1 tomato, sliced,
1 teaspoon ground flaxseed	or 1 green bell pepper, sliced
2 slices whole-wheat bread, toasted	½ cup orange juice

1. Scramble the whole egg and egg whites in a bowl. Add ground flaxseed to the mixture.

2. Fry in a nonstick skillet spritzed with vegetable oil spray, and dump onto the toast.

3. Add bacon and tomatoes, peppers, or other vegetables of your choice.

Makes: 1 serving

Per serving: 399 calories, 31 g protein, 46 g carbohydrates, 11 g fat (3 g saturated fat), 900 mg sodium, 6 g fiber

---

ABS DIET SUCCESS STORY

"I Turned Flab into Muscle!"

Name: John Betson

Age: 25

Height: 5'10"

Starting weight: 180

Six weeks later: 165

Fathers pass down a lot of things to their sons, but John Betson inherited one thing from his dad that he didn't want: flabby breast tissue. "I've always had flab on my chest, and since I was a kid, I've had to work hard to keep from looking like the Dolly Parton of the gym," Betson says.

High school football took care of it for a while, but graduation and a 60-hour-a-week desk job added roundness in two places he didn't want—his gut and his pecs. Fifteen pounds overweight, Betson decided to get back in shape. "I wanted to make sure I looked good for my wife," he says. "I didn't want to give her a reason to look elsewhere."

Breakfast Bacon Burger (number of powerfoods: 4)

1 Thomas' Honey Wheat English Muffin	1 slice low-fat American cheese
½ teaspoon trans fat–free margarine	1 slice Canadian bacon
1 egg	Vegetables of choice

1. Split the muffin, toast it, and add margarine.

2. Break the egg in a microwavable dish, prick the yolk with a toothpick, and cover the dish with plastic wrap.

3. Microwave on high for 30 seconds. Let stand for 30 seconds. Add cheese, egg, and Canadian bacon to the muffin, then nuke for 20 seconds.

4. Add vegetables to taste.

Makes: 1 serving

Per serving: 300 calories, 22 g protein, 28 g carbohydrates, 11 g fat (3.5 g saturated fat), 868 mg sodium, 3 g fiber

---

The first week on the Abs Diet was the toughest because it was so counterintuitive. Betson was used to eating only two meals a day. He'd eat a banana and a pack of crackers for lunch. Then, armed with the feeling that he hadn't eaten much during the day, he'd load up on massive helpings of meat loaf and pizza for dinner. But the Abs Diet required him to eat often—up to six times a day. "I felt fat at first because I was eating so much, but after the first week, I loved it. I loved the food, and I loved feeling stronger and more energetic," he says.

He also lifted 3 days a week and did cardio work 3 days a week, which resulted in a dramatic change in body composition. He lost 15 pounds and decreased his percentage of body fat from 23 to 16 percent. "You can see more muscle. You can see my abs," he says.

What's even more amazing is that at the same time Betson started the Abs Diet, he quit smoking—a time when most people gain weight.

Down from a 36-inch waist to a 32- or 33-inch waist, Betson says the biggest change he's felt is actually internal. He says, "Confidence—having more confidence—is the biggest improvement I've seen."

The I-Haven't-Had-My-Coffee-Yet Sandwich
(number of powerfoods: 3)

1½ teaspoons low-fat cream cheese

1 whole-wheat pita, halved to make 2 pockets

2 slices turkey or ham

Lettuce or green vegetable

1. Spread cream cheese in the pockets of the pita.
2. Stuff with meat and vegetables.
3. Put in mouth. Chew and swallow.

Makes: 1 serving

Per serving: 225 calories, 10 grams protein, 42 g carbohydrates, 3g fat (1 g saturated fat), 430 mg sodium, 6 g fiber

Honey, I Shrunk My Gut (number of powerfoods: 5)

1 cup 1 percent milk

¾ cup plain instant oatmeal

½ cup blueberries or blackberries

1 tablespoon chopped walnuts or pecans

1 teaspoon honey

1 teaspoon ground flaxseed

Pinch of ground cinnamon

Mix the milk and oatmeal in a microwavable bowl. Microwave for 2 minutes or until thick. Stir in the remaining ingredients.

Makes: 1 serving

Per serving: 340 calories, 15 grams protein, 52g carbohydrates, 10g fat (2.5 g saturated fat), 190 mg sodium, 6 g fiber

► **FROM THE NEW ABS DIET COOKBOOK!**

Flapjacks with Chocolate Chips (number of powerfoods: 4)

¾ cup whole-wheat flour	1 tablespoon brown sugar
1 tablespoon baking powder	1 teaspoon vanilla extract
1 teaspoon salt	2 eggs, lightly beaten
1½ cups 2 percent milk	½ cup chocolate chips
1 cup plain instant oatmeal	

1. Mix the flour, baking powder, and salt in a small bowl. Mix the milk, oatmeal, sugar, and vanilla in a large bowl. Stir in the eggs and then add the dry ingredients, a little at a time. Stir in the chocolate chips.

2. Coat a griddle or nonstick skillet with cooking spray and heat over medium-high heat. Using a measuring cup, pour about ¼ cup of batter onto the hot surface for each pancake. When the edges of the pancakes are cooked and little bubbles form in the middle, flip the pancakes over. Cook until golden brown.

Makes: *about 10 pancakes*

Per pancake: *140 calories, 5 g protein, 20 g carbohydrates, 5 g fat (2.5 g saturated fat), 430 mg sodium, 2 g fiber*

Breakfast with Barbie (number of powerfoods: 3)

1 packet instant grits	1 tablespoon low-fat shredded Cheddar cheese
4 frozen shrimp, defrosted and chopped	1 dollop barbecue sauce

Prepare the grits according to package directions. Add the shrimp and cheese, stirring well to blend. Top with the barbecue sauce.

Makes: *1 serving*

Per serving: *167 calories, 9 g protein, 31 g carbohydrates, 1 g fat (0 g saturated fat), 731 mg sodium, 2 g fiber*

The 'Bama Bowl (number of powerfoods: 4)

1 packet instant grits	2 strips beef jerky, finely diced
1 teaspoon ground flaxseed	1 tablespoon low-fat shredded Cheddar cheese

Prepare the grits according to package directions. Add the flaxseed, jerky, and cheese, stirring well to blend.

Makes: 1 serving

Per serving: 199 calories, 11 g protein, 26 g carbohydrates, 6 g fat (2 g saturated fat), 786 mg sodium, 3 g fiber

▶ FROM THE NEW ABS DIET COOKBOOK!

Grilled Banana Sandwiches (number of powerfoods: 3)

1 large banana	1 tablespoon honey
1½ tablespoons low-fat whipped cream cheese	Pinch of salt
1½ tablespoons peanut butter	4 slices whole-grain bread

1. Cut off one-quarter of the banana and mash in a bowl with a fork; stir in the cream cheese, peanut butter, honey and salt. Spread over 2 bread slices.

2. Coat a large skillet with cooking spray and place over medium-high heat. Slice the remaining banana in half lengthwise and then in half crosswise. Place the banana halves in the pan and cook until caramelized. Arrange the bananas over the cream cheese and top with the remaining bread.

3. Wipe out the skillet, add a spritz more cooking spray, and place over medium heat. Add the sandwiches and cook until browned on each side.

Makes: 2 servings

Per serving: 320 calories, 11 g protein, 50 g carbohydrates, 10 g fat (2 g saturated fat), 320 mg sodium, 6 g fiber

Abs Diet Lunches

IN THE MIDDLE of a workday, drive-throughs and pizza stands can be more tempting than that coworker with the great glutes. Be strong! You can still follow the eating plan no matter where you are. Grilled chicken and chili are usually good options. In sit-down situations, you can also order smartly without getting tripped up by the quesadilla special. Some good combinations include a salad with grilled chicken or salmon, vegetables, almonds or other nuts, and a sprinkling of balsamic vinegar and olive oil. You can also order a piece of lean meat—either on whole-grain bread or by itself—with a side of vegetables. Ask for salsa or a small side of olive oil for dipping. If you bring your lunch or eat it at home, these are some other options.

► FROM THE NEW ABS DIET COOKBOOK!

The Johnny Apple Cheese Sandwich (number of powerfoods: 3)

2   slices 7-grain bread

2   teaspoons light mayonnaise

1   teaspoon Dijon mustard

2   slices low-fat Swiss cheese

1   Red Delicious apple, halved and thinly sliced

1   tablespoon chopped walnuts

1. Preheat a toaster oven to 350°F.

2. Spread 1 bread slice with mayonnaise and the other with mustard. Top each with cheese.

3. Place on a tray and put into the toaster oven until the cheese has melted. Top 1 bread slice with the apple and sprinkle with the walnuts. Press the sandwich halves together.

Makes: 1 serving

*Per serving: 440 calories, 19 g; **Carbohydrates:** 46 g carbohydrates, 21 g fat (7 g saturated fat), 500 mg sodium, 8 g fiber*

The I-Am-Not-Eating-Salad Salad (number of powerfoods: 4)

2 ounces grilled chicken

1 cup romaine lettuce

1 tomato, chopped

1 small green bell pepper, chopped

1 medium carrot, chopped

3 tablespoons Italian 94 percent fat-free Italian dressing or 1 teaspoon of olive oil

1 tablespoon grated Parmesan cheese

1 tablespoon ground flaxseed

1. Chop the chicken into small pieces.

2. Mix all the ingredients together, and store in the fridge. Eat on multigrain bread or by itself.

Makes: 1 serving

Per serving: 248 calories, 16 g protein, 33 g carbohydrates, 8 g fat (2 g saturated fat), 875 mg sodium, 10 g fiber

||||||||||||||||||||||||||||||||||||||||||||||||||||||||||||||||||||||||||||||||||||||||||||||||||||||||

6 Foods with Surprising Health Benefits

1. Coconut. It contains more saturated fat than butter, but more than half of that is lauric acid. An analysis of 60 studies in the *American Journal of Clinical Nutrition* concludes that while lauric acid increases bad cholesterol, it boosts the good so significantly it may actually decrease your risk of cardiovascular disease.

2. Pork Chops. Purdue University researchers found that a 6-ounce serving daily of the other white meat helped people preserve their muscle while losing weight.

3. Mushrooms. Mushrooms create metabolites during digestion that boost immunity and prevent cancer growth, according to researchers in the Netherlands.

4. Red-Pepper Flakes. A Dutch study shows that by consuming about half a teaspoon of red pepper 30 minutes prior to a meal, you can reduce calorie intake by 16 percent. Plus, capsaicin—the active ingredient in hot peppers—may help kill cancer cells.

5. Full-Fat Cheese. You know that dairy is one of the 12 Abs Diet Powerfoods, but full-fat cheese? Yes. It's an excellent source of casein protein, one of the best muscle-building nutrients you can eat.

6. Vinegar. Sprinkle it on your sandwich. Scientists in Sweden discovered that when people ate 2 tablespoons of vinegar with a meal high in carbohydrates, their blood sugar was 23 percent lower than when they skipped the antioxidant-loaded liquid.

Guilt-Free BLT (number of powerfoods: 3)

¾ tablespoon fat-free mayonnaise	2 ounces roasted turkey breast, diced
1 whole-wheat tortilla	2 slices tomato
2 slices turkey bacon, cooked	2 leaves lettuce

1. Smear the mayo on the tortilla.

2. Line the middle of the tortilla with the bacon and top with turkey breast, tomato, and lettuce.

3. Roll it tightly into a tube.

Makes: 1 serving

Per serving: 206 calories, 17 g protein, 26 g carbohydrates, 7 g fat (2 g saturated fat), 1,270 mg sodium, 3 g fiber

Guac and Roll (number of powerfoods: 4)

1 can (6 ounces) light oil-packed tuna	1 tablespoon light mayonnaise
⅔ cup guacamole	1 teaspoon ground flaxseed
¼ cup chopped tomatoes	2 6-inch whole-wheat hoagie rolls
1 teaspoon lemon juice	

1. Combine the first six ingredients in a bowl and blend thoroughly with a fork.

2. Split the rolls in half, and fill each half with ¼ cup of the mixture.

Makes: 2 servings

Per serving: 606 calories, 36 g protein, 58 g carbohydrates, 28 g fat (5 g saturated fat), 942 mg sodium, 13 g fiber

Hot Tuna (number of powerfoods: 4)

½ cup chopped celery

1 onion, chopped

½ cup shredded, reduced-fat mozzarella cheese

½ cup reduced-fat cottage cheese

1 can (6 ounces) water-packed tuna, drained and flaked

¼ cup reduced-fat mayonnaise

1 tablespoon lemon juice

3 whole-wheat English muffins, split in half

1. Preheat your oven to 350°F. In a large nonstick skillet over low heat, cook the celery and onion until softened. Add the cheeses, tuna, mayo, and lemon juice to the skillet, and cook the mixture just long enough to warm it up.

2. Spread one-sixth of the mixture on each English muffin half. Put the muffin halves on a baking sheet, and bake for 10 minutes.

Makes: 2 servings

Per serving: 628 calories, 50 g protein, 54 g carbohydrates, 24 g fat (6 g saturated fat), 1,300 mg sodium, 8 g fiber

‖‖‖

When You're Out

AT THE	EAT THIS	NOT THAT
Ballpark	Hot dog with sauerkraut, 16-ounce light beer, soft pretzel: 750 calories, 16 g fat, 18 g protein	Chili dog, 16-ounce regular beer, cheese nachos: 1,174 calories, 60 g fat, 34 g protein
Steakhouse	6-ounce grilled top round, baked sweet potato, ear of corn with pat of butter: 688 calories, 22 g fat, 60 g protein	6-ounce rib eye, 2 cups fries, ½ cup broccoli with cheese: 1,153 calories, 52 g fat, 62 g protein
Sushi bar	1 California roll, 6 salmon nigiri, 1 cup miso soup: 804 calories, 10 g fat, 28 g protein	1 orange roll, 1 spicy shrimp roll, 1½ cups salad with ginger dressing: 1,262 calories, 32 g fat, 59 g protein

Yo Soup for You (number of powerfoods: 3)

½ pound chicken breast

1 cup chopped onion

1 teaspoon olive oil

2 cloves garlic, minced

6 cups low-sodium chicken stock

1 cup canned navy beans, drained

½ cup minced carrots

1 cup corn

2 tablespoons chopped basil or parsley

¼ teaspoon ground black pepper

½ cup canned peeled tomatoes

1. In a large saucepan over low heat, cook the chicken and onion in the oil for about 10 minutes, or until the onion is golden brown. Add the garlic and cook for 1 minute.

2. Add the stock, beans, and carrots. Bring to a boil. Add the corn, basil, black pepper, and tomatoes (with juice). Cook for 15 minutes.

Makes: 4 servings

Per serving: 260 calories, 27 g protein, 30 g carbohydrates, 5 g fat (1 g saturated fat), 602 mg sodium, 6 g fiber

Nice-to-Meat-You Sandwich (number of powerfoods: 3)

2 slices whole-wheat bread

2 ounces sliced roast beef

2 inner leaves romaine lettuce

1 teaspoon low-fat mayonnaise

1 ounce fat-free American cheese

Stack everything up into a sandwich.

Makes: 1 serving

Per serving: 380 calories, 28 g protein, 32 g carbohydrates, 17 g fat (6 g saturated fat), 811 mg sodium, 4 g fiber

Hurry Curry (number of powerfoods: 3)

½ cup fat-free plain yogurt

½ cup fat-free mayonnaise

3 tablespoons finely chopped onions

1 teaspoon ginger

1 teaspoon curry powder

1 pound boneless, skinless chicken breast, cut into ½-inch strips

1 teaspoon paprika

½ teaspoon ground black pepper

2 cups cooked brown rice

1. In a small bowl, mix the yogurt, mayonnaise, onion, ginger, and curry powder.

2. Place the chicken in a medium bowl. Sprinkle with the paprika and pepper. Toss until coated.

3. In a nonstick skillet over medium heat, cook the chicken for 4 to 5 minutes. Stir in the yogurt mixture. Cook, stirring, for 2 minutes. Serve over the rice.

Makes: 2 servings

Per serving: 598 calories, 61 g protein, 69 g carbohydrates, 7 g fat (1 g saturated fat), 704 mg sodium, 6 g fiber

Popeye and Olive Oil (number of powerfoods: 4)

1½ cups chopped baby spinach leaves

1½ cups chopped romaine lettuce

3 slices prosciutto, chopped

⅓ cup mandarin orange slices

⅓ cup sliced strawberries

2 tablespoons diced red onion

For dressing:

1½ teaspoons olive oil

1 tablespoon red wine vinegar

½ clove garlic, crushed

⅛ teaspoon black pepper

In a bowl, mix together all of the ingredients. Store in the fridge until you are ready to eat.

Makes: 1 serving

Per serving: 238 calories, 9 g protein, 23 g carbohydrates, 14 g fat (4 g saturated fat), 450 mg sodium, 6 g fiber

The Two Chicks (number of powerfoods: 4)

3 cups mixed greens

⅓ cup garbanzo beans (chickpeas), rinsed and drained

½ cup diced precooked chicken breast

½ cup diced ready-made roasted red peppers

1 teaspoon ground flaxseed

For dressing:

1½ tablespoons low-fat ranch dressing, such as Hidden Valley

2 cans (16 ounces) whole tomatoes

1 jar (20 ounces) spaghetti sauce

2 tablespoons Italian seasoning

1 package (1 pound) whole-wheat spaghetti

In a large bowl, mix together all of the ingredients. Store in the fridge until you are ready to eat.

Makes: *1 serving*

Per serving: *391 calories, 41 g protein, 27 g carbohydrates, 12 g fat (2 g saturated fat), 884 mg sodium, 8 g fiber*

The Melon Banquet (number of powerfoods: 4)

3 cups mixed greens

⅓ cup cubed watermelon

½ cup cubed cantaloupe

2 tablespoons grated carrot

1 ounce smoked salmon, chopped

1 tablespoon pine nuts

1 teaspoon chopped mint

For dressing:

1½ teaspoons olive oil

2 teaspoons balsamic vinegar

1 teaspoon lemon juice

In a bowl, mix together all of the ingredients. Store in the fridge until you are ready to eat.

Makes: *1 serving*

Per serving: *274 calories, 11 g protein, 20 g carbohydrates, 19 g fat (2 g saturated fat), 635 mg sodium, 5 g fiber*

Abs Diet Dinners

DINNER IS THE place where most of us wind down and pork up. That's because we spend the day serving others. By dinnertime, we're hungry to have some of our own demands met. On this plan, you'll have already fueled up four times before dinner, so you'll feel pleasantly hungry, not ravenous. These meals give you the taste of sin—without the actual guilt.

Mas Macho Meatballs (number of powerfoods: 3)

1 pound extra-lean ground beef	1 tablespoon ground flaxseed or whey powder
½ cup crushed saltine crackers	1 jar (16 ounces) tomato sauce
1 large onion, diced	4 whole-wheat hoagie rolls
1 clove garlic, minced	½ cup reduced-fat mozzarella cheese, shredded

1. Mix the beef, crackers, onion, garlic, and flaxseed or whey powder into golf ball–size meatballs.

2. In a nonstick skillet over medium heat, cook the meatballs until browned all the way around. Drain the fat from the skillet, and add the tomato sauce.

3. While the mixture is warming, use a fork to scoop out some of the bread in the rolls to form shallow trenches. Spoon the meatballs and sauce into each trench, and sprinkle with shredded mozzarella, and top with the top half of the roll.

Makes: 4 servings

Per serving: 569 calories, 38 g protein, 65 g carbohydrates, 19 g fat (6 g saturated fat), 1,341 mg sodium, 10 g fiber

▶ FROM THE NEW ABS DIET COOKBOOK!

A Thinner Mexican Dinner (number of powerfoods: 5)

For meat:

- ¾ pound lean ground beef (90 percent lean or higher)
- 2 cloves garlic, minced
- 1 can (15.5 ounces) black beans, rinsed and drained
- 1 tablespoon chili powder
- ¼ teaspoon cayenne
- ⅓ cup water

For dressing:

- 4 medium tomatoes, diced
- 2 tablespoons extra-virgin olive oil
- 2 tablespoons lime juice
- ½ teaspoon salt
- ¼ teaspoon black pepper

For salad:

- 2 romaine lettuce hearts, chopped
- ½ cup shredded reduced-fat Cheddar cheese
- 2 ounces baked corn tortilla chips (about 32 chips)

1. Heat a large skillet over medium-high heat. Add the beef and cook, breaking up the pieces with a wooden spoon, until no longer pink. Add the garlic and beans and cook for 2 minutes more. Add the chili powder, cayenne, and water and stir until well combined and some but not all of the liquid has been absorbed. Remove from the heat and allow the mixture to cool slightly.

2. Mix the dressing ingredients in a bowl.

3. Divide the lettuce among dinner plates, top with the beef mixture, and sprinkle with cheese. Spoon the dressing over each salad and crush tortilla chips on top.

Makes: 4 servings

Per serving: 440 calories, 32 g protein, 43 g carbohydrates, 19 g fat (6 g saturated fat), 870 mg sodium, 11 g fiber

Bodacious Brazilian Chicken (number of powerfoods: 2)

1 lemon

1 lime

1 tablespoon ground flaxseed

1 can (8 ounces) tomato sauce

1 can (6 ounces) frozen orange juice concentrate

1½ cloves garlic, minced

1 teaspoon dried Italian seasoning

4 boneless, skinless chicken breast halves

1 teaspoon hot pepper salsa

¾ cup chunky salsa

1. Grate the zest of the lemon and lime into a resealable bag. Squeeze the juice from both fruits into the bag, and throw out the pulp and the seeds.

2. Mix in everything else except the chicken and salsa.

3. Drop in the chicken, reseal the bag, and refrigrate for a few hours.

4. Grill the chicken, turning and basting with marinade a few times, for 10 to 15 minutes or until the center is no longer pink. Serve with salsa.

Makes: 4 servings

Per serving: 205 calories, 29 g protein, 18 g carbohydrates, 2 g fat (0.5 g saturated fat), 726 mg sodium, 3 g fiber

Chile-Peppered Steak (number of powerfoods: 4)

1 tablespoon olive oil

2 carrots, sliced

1 cup chopped broccoli

2 jalapeño peppers, sliced

2 cayenne peppers, sliced

12 ounces lean sirloin steak, sliced thin

¼ cup Hunan stir-fry sauce

4 cups cooked brown rice

1. Heat the oil in a nonstick skillet over high heat. Toss in the carrots and broccoli, and cook until tender.

2. Add the peppers and beef, and continue cooking until meat is done.

3. Add sauce, and serve over rice.

Makes: 4 servings

Per serving: 485 calories, 32 g protein, 57 g carbohydrates, 14 g fat (3.5 g saturated fat), 224 mg sodium, 6 g fiber

▶ FROM THE NEW ABS DIET COOKBOOK!

Tuna with Wasabi (number of powerfoods: 2)

2 tablespoons reduced-sodium soy sauce

2 tablespoons rice vinegar

1 tablespoon sugar

½ teaspoon toasted sesame oil

½ teaspoon ground ginger

1½ pounds tuna steaks

¼ cup reduced-fat sour cream

½ teaspoon wasabi paste

1. Mix the soy sauce, vinegar, sugar, oil, and ginger in glass baking dish. Add the tuna steaks, turning to coat. Cover and allow to marinate in the refrigerator for 30 minutes, turning twice. Mix the sour cream and wasabi in a small bowl.

2. Coat a grill pan with cooking spray. Remove the tuna from the dish and discard the marinade. Place the steaks on the hot grill pan. Cook for 6 minutes, turning once, for medium-rare. Serve with the wasabi sauce.

Makes: 6 servings

Per serving: 194 calories, 27 g protein, 4 g carbohydrates, 7 g fat (2 g saturated fat), 227 mg sodium, 0 g fiber

Philadelphia Fryers (number of powerfoods: 3)

1 medium onion, sliced

1 small red bell pepper, sliced

1 small green bell pepper, sliced

⅔ cup medium or hot salsa

4 multigrain hoagie rolls

¾ pound roast beef, thinly sliced

½ cup grated reduced-fat Cheddar cheese

1. In a nonstick skillet over medium heat, cook the onion and peppers until tender. Add the salsa and heat until warm.

2. Construct the sandwiches with the buns, roast beef, onions, peppers, and cheese, then warm them in the microwave for 1 to 2 minutes on high, until the cheese starts to melt.

Makes: 4 sandwiches

Calories per sandwich: 558 calories, 35 g protein, 40 g carbohydrates, 28 g fat (12.5 g saturated fat), 653 mg sodium, 4 g fiber

Chili Con Turkey (number of powerfoods: 4)

1 pound ground turkey

1 can (14 ounces) Mexican-style diced tomatoes

1 can (15 ounces) black beans, rinsed and drained

1 can (14 ounces) whole-kernel sweet corn, drained

1 package (1½ ounces) dried chili mix

1 tablespoon ground flaxseed

¼ cup water

1 cup cooked rice

1. In a large nonstick skillet over medium-high heat, brown the turkey.

2. Add everything else but the rice, and cook over low heat for 10 minutes. Serve over rice.

Makes: 4 servings

Per serving: 407 calories, 30 g protein, 52 g carbohydrates, 11 g fat (3 g saturated fat), 1,578 mg sodium, 9 g fiber

Chicken à la King Kong (number of powerfoods: 3)

2 tablespoons olive oil

½ onion, finely chopped

1 teaspoon flour

2 tablespoons water

4 teaspoons chili powder

1 pound chicken breast tenders

1 cup spaghetti sauce

9 ounces cooked whole-wheat spaghetti

1. Heat the oil in a nonstick skillet over medium-high heat. Add the onion and cook for 1 minute, until browned. In a small bowl, mix the flour and water.

2. Add chicken, chili powder, sauce, and flour mixture to skillet. Stir. Simmer uncovered for 10 minutes. Serve over cooked spaghetti.

Makes: 4 servings

Per serving: 320 calories, 31 g protein, 26 g carbohydrates, 10 g fat (2 g saturated fat), 360 mg sodium, 5 g fiber

Salmon Rushdie (number of powerfoods: 5)

2 tablespoons olive oil

1 tablespoon lemon juice

¼ teaspoon salt

¼ teaspoon ground black pepper

1 tablespoon ground flaxseed

1 clove garlic

4 6-ounce salmon fillets

Green vegetable of choice

1 cup cooked rice

1. In a baking dish, combine the oil, lemon juice, salt, pepper, flaxseed, and garlic. Add the fish, coat well, cover, and refrigerate for 15 minutes.

2. Preheat your oven to 450°F. Line a baking sheet with foil, and coat it with cooking spray. Remove the fish from the marinade, and place the fish skin side down on the baking sheet.

3. Bake for 9 to 12 minutes. Serve with a green vegetable and rice.

Makes: 4 servings

Per serving: 411 calories, 40 g protein, 15 g carbohydrates, 20 g fat (3 g saturated fat), 231 mg sodium, 1 g fiber

Spaghettaboudit! (number of powerfoods: 3)

¾ pound extra-lean ground beef

1½ onions, chopped

1 green bell pepper, chopped

2 cloves garlic, minced

1 cup sliced mushrooms

2 cans (16 ounces) whole tomatoes

1 jar (20 ounces) spaghetti sauce

2 tablespoons Italian seasoning

1 package (1 pound) whole-wheat spaghetti

1. In a large saucepan over medium-high heat, cook the meat until browned. Drain the fat from the meat.

2. Add onion, green pepper, and garlic, and cook until tender. Pour in mushrooms, tomatoes (with juice), sauce, and seasoning, and stir everything together. Simmer. In a separate pot, cook the spaghetti according to the package directions.

3. Serve ½ cup of sauce over 1 cup of spaghetti.

Makes: 4 servings

Per serving: 400 calories, 28 protein, 50 g carbohydrates, 12 g fat (4 g saturated fat), 798 mg sodium, 10 g fiber

Three Amigos Chili (number of powerfoods: 5)

1 tablespoon extra-virgin olive oil	1 can (10.5 ounces) kidney beans, rinsed and drained
1 small onion, diced	1 can (14 ounces) low-sodium chicken broth
1 pound ground turkey breast	
1 can (14.5 ounces) diced tomatoes with jalapeños	½ teaspoon salt
	½ teaspoon ground cumin
1 can (10.5 ounces) chickpeas, rinsed and drained	⅛ teaspoon ground cinnamon
	Hot sauce
1 can (10.5 ounces) black beans, rinsed and drained	

1. Heat the oil in a large saucepan over medium-low heat. Add the onion and cook until soft, about 3 to 5 minutes.

2. Add the turkey and cook, breaking up the pieces with a wooden spoon, until browned, about 5 minutes.

3. Add the tomatoes with juice, beans, broth, and spices. Stir and bring to a boil, then reduce the heat and simmer for 20 minutes. Serve with hot sauce.

Makes 6 servings

Per serving: 293 calories, 31 g protein, 32 g carbohydrates, 5 g fat (0 g saturated fat), 788 mg sodium, 11 g fiber

▶ FROM THE NEW ABS DIET COOKBOOK!

Maria's Portobellos (number of powerfoods: 1)

2 tablespoons extra-virgin olive oil	1 clove garlic, minced
	1 pound large portobello mushrooms
2 tablespoons balsamic vinegar	
	Salt and pepper

1. Mix the oil, vinegar, and garlic in a large bowl. Add the mushrooms and gently toss to coat. Allow the mushrooms to marinate for 30 minutes.

2. Remove from the marinade and grill, roast, or broil until golden brown. Season with salt and pepper.

Makes: 6 servings

Per serving: 70 calories, 2 g protein, 5 g carbohydrates, 5 g fat (0.5 g saturated fat), 200 mg sodium, 1 g fiber

Abs Diet Snacks

MOST DIET PLANS portray snacking as a failure. I want you to think of snacking as exactly the opposite—as a key to success! But the secret to effective snacking is doing so at the optimum time—about 2 hours before you're scheduled to eat your next meal. That'll be enough time to head off hunger pangs and keep you full enough to avoid a meltdown at mealtime. You have a lot of flexibility in what you use to snack. You could have a portion of a leftover from dinner, a sandwich, a smoothie, or a combination of some of the 12 Abs Diet Powerfoods. To make it easier, pick one food from column A and one from column B. That will ensure your satiety.

A		B	
PROTEIN	**DAIRY**	**FRUIT OR VEGETABLE**	**COMPLEX CARBOHYDRATE**
2 teaspoons reduced-fat peanut butter	8 ounces low-fat yogurt	1 ounce raisins	1 or 2 slices whole-grain bread
1 ounce almonds	1 cup 1 percent milk or chocolate milk	Raw vegetables (celery, baby carrots, broccoli), unlimited	1 bowl oatmeal or high-fiber cereal
3 slices low-sodium deli turkey breast	$\frac{3}{4}$ cup low-fat ice cream	1$\frac{1}{2}$ cup berries	
3 slices deli roast beef	1$\frac{1}{2}$ slices fat-free cheese	4 ounces cantaloupe	
	1 stick string cheese	1 large orange	
		1 can (11.5 ounces) low-sodium V8 juice	

Abs Diet Desserts

IF YOU HAVE always enjoyed something sweet after dinner, don't deny yourself now. Just be smart about it. Use dessert as your third snack of the day, either right after dinner or a little later in the evening. The following recipes appear decadent, but they keep calories and fat in check, thanks to certain power-foods. That's not to say you can have seconds. Keep your portions small and you'll be able to enjoy sweets now and then without sabotaging your weight-loss efforts.

▶ FROM THE NEW ABS DIET COOKBOOK!

Coffee with Dessert (number of powerfoods: 2)

1½ cups ricotta cheese

½ cup light cream cheese

½ cup sugar

3 tablespoons cocoa

1 egg yolk

1 teaspoon vanilla

3 egg whites

⅓ cup sugar

¾ cup strong, prepared coffee

3 tablespoons coffee-flavored liqueur

16 ladyfinger cookies

1. In a food processor, combine the ricotta cheese, cream cheese, sugar, cocoa, egg yolk and vanilla until smooth; transfer to a bowl.

2. Beat egg whites in a bowl until soft peaks form. Gradually add sugar and beat until stiff peaks form. Fold the egg whites into the ricotta mixture.

3. Combine the coffee and the liqueur in a small bowl.

4. Arrange half of the cookies in the bottom of a 9-inch square baking dish that you've sprayed with nonstick spray. Sprinkle with half of the coffee mixture. Spread half of the ricotta mixture on top. Repeat one more layer. Cover and chill overnight.

Makes: 16 servings

Per serving: 150 calories, 6 g protein, 21 g carbohydrates, 5 g fat (2 g saturated fat), 102 mg sodium, 0 g fiber

Yogi Pops (number of powerfoods: 1)

1 six-pack (4-ounce cups) of your favorite flavor of reduced-fat yogurt

6 Popsicle sticks

Pierce each yogurt pack with a stick. Freeze.

Makes: *6 servings*

Per serving: *118 calories, 4 g protein, 24 g carbohydrates, 1 g fat (0 g saturated), 59 mg sodium, 0 g fiber*

Berried Alive (number of powerfoods: 5)

1 cup each frozen blueberries, strawberries, and raspberries

¼ cup balsamic vinegar

1 teaspoon dried basil

1 scoop reduced-fat ice cream

Sprinkle of sugar

Place berries, vinegar, basil, and sugar in a plastic container. Shake well to mix, then store in the fridge (should last for up to a week). Top a scoop of your favorite reduced-fat ice cream with ½ cup of berry mixture.

Makes: *6 servings*

Per serving: *262 calories, 6 g protein, 43 g carbohydrates, 8 g fat (5 g saturated fat), 84 mg sodium, 3 g fiber*

Bananacicles (number of powerfoods: 1)

4 Popsicle sticks

2 bananas, peeled and cut in half crosswise

½ cup chocolate sauce (the kind that forms a shell)

4 tablespoons unsalted peanuts, diced.

Put a Popsicle stick into the cut end of each banana piece. Pour chocolate sauce over bananas until they're completely coated. Roll chocolate-coated bananas in peanuts. Freeze.

Makes: *4 servings*

Per serving: *318 calories, 4 g protein, 32 g carbohydrates, 22 g fat (9 g saturated fat), 21 mg sodium, 4 g fiber*

Piece of Cake (number of powerfoods: 2)

2 slices ready-made frozen pound cake

3 strawberries, sliced

2 teaspoons chocolate hazelnut spread (such as Nutella)

Slice cake and place on a medium-hot grill pan. Grill for 1 to 2 minutes per side. Spread with chocolate hazelnut spread and berries, then top with another slice of cake, like a sandwich.

Makes: 2 servings

Per serving: 340 calories, 6 g protein, 46 g carbohydrates, 15 g fat (7 g saturated fat), 283 mg sodium, 2 g fiber

||||||||||||||||||||||||||||||||||||||||||||||||||||||||||||||||||||||||||||||||||||||||||||||||||||||

What's a 100-Calorie Portion?

Proteins

2 ounces or 2 slices low-fat American or Cheddar cheese

2 slices bacon

2 ounces chicken (no skin)

2 small eggs

1½ cups fat-free milk

1 cup 1 percent milk

½ ounce roasted peanuts

2 ounces pork

2 ounces salmon or tuna

4 ounces (about 15) shrimp

Fats

1 tablespoon butter

2 teaspoons olive or corn oil

1 tablespoon mayo

1 tablespoon peanut butter

Carbs

¾ cup All-Bran cereal

1 large apple

1 medium banana

2 cups (about 50) green beans

½ cup corn

¾ cup plain oatmeal

1 ounce pasta

½ medium baked potato

20 medium strawberries

8 teaspoons sugar

2½ slices low-calorie wheat bread

Muscle Muffins (number of powerfoods: 3)

1 banana, mashed	1 scoop vanilla whey protein powder
1 apple, shredded	
½ cup unsweetened applesauce	1 cup whole-grain pastry flour
	3 tablespoons brown sugar
¼ cup chopped walnuts	2 teaspoons baking powder

Preheat the oven to 350°F. Coat a nonstick muffin pan with cooking spray. Mix all the ingredients. Spoon into the muffin cups. Bake for 20 minutes or until a toothpick inserted into the center of a muffin comes out clean.

Makes: 12 muffins

Per serving: 90 calories, 3 g protein, 15 g carbohydrates, 2 g fat (0 g saturated), 85 mg sodium, 2 g fiber

▶ **FROM THE NEW ABS DIET COOKBOOK!**

Whip-It-Good Banana Split (number of powerfoods: 3)

2 cups fat-free milk	½ cup fat-free whipped topping
1 package (4 servings) Jell-o Instant Sugar-free Chocolate Pudding Mix	1 tablespoon chopped peanuts
2 ripe bananas, sliced	4 bing cherries, stem on (optional)

Whisk together the milk and pudding mix for about 2 minutes. Spoon half into dessert dishes. Top with bananas and then the remaining pudding. Divide the whipped topping, peanuts, and cherries among the dishes. Let stand until set, about 5 minutes.

Makes: 4 servings

Per serving: 130 caloires, 5 g protein, 24 g carbohydrates, 1.5 g fat (0 g saturated), 75 mg sodium, 2 g fiber

Chapter 10

FITTING THE NEW ABS DIET INTO EVERYDAY LIFE

How This Simple Eating Plan Makes Your Life Simpler, Too

I N PREVIOUS CHAPTERS, I outlined why the New Abs Diet works—and will work for you, for life. I gave an overview of the science and fed you some nifty terms like glycemic index and basal metabolism. And I listed a whole eating plan complete with meals, snacks, and simple recipes.

But I also explained why most other diet plans are the nutritional equivalent of that tape recorder in *Mission: Impossible*—programmed to self-destruct in 5 seconds, or 5 weeks, or 5 years. Most diets just aren't designed to last over the long haul, or they're so complicated and restrictive that you'd have to quit your day job and disown half your friends in order to follow them to the letter. Many diets fail because they require us to work too hard and ignore the fact that we're already working too hard. What most of us feel, every day, is that our worlds are on the verge of spinning out of control. And what we want is to take back control: to take control of our lives, our careers, our relationships, our bodies, our diets, ourselves.

That's why I want to take a break at this point and demonstrate for you how easily the New Abs Diet fits into a busy lifestyle and how adopting its simple eating strategies can take a lot of the work, stress, and hassle out of everyday life. To do that, I've decided to give you a quick profile of a day in the life of a typical hardworking guy. Let's call him Joe.

A Day in the Life of Joe

6:30 a.m. Joe wakes up, staggers out to the kitchen, and starts the coffeepot. While the coffee's brewing, he pulls a mug out of a cabinet and fills it with fat-free or 1 percent milk. He drinks the milk down until there's about $\frac{1}{8}$ cup left, then pours in the coffee.[1] Then he grabs the papers and flips through them quickly, stopping at the obituaries just in case he died the night before and nobody told him.

7 a.m. Joe turns on the morning talk shows, and while the goofy smiling weatherman tells him what's in store for the day, he takes some ice, some yogurt, a spoonful each of whey protein and ground flaxseed, plus some leftover fruit and maybe some lime juice or orange juice or whatever else happens to be laying around the kitchen, and throws the whole menagerie into a blender. He buzzes that into oblivion for 30 seconds, pours some into a glass, and pours the rest of it into a thermos, which he will carry to his office.[2]

8 a.m. Having showered, shaved, and dressed, Joe leaves his house and walks to work, which takes about 35 minutes. Before he goes to the office, he stops at a deli and grabs a little packet of almonds and an apple, which he sticks in his desk. He sticks his Thermos of smoothie into the fridge in the office kitchen. Then he goes through his work—returns phone calls, answers e-mail, and the like.

1. A blast of low-fat protein and calcium gives you an immediate metabolic boost and helps ensure you get your daily allotment of calcium and vitamin D. The coffee cup ritual is just a good reminder to have that glass of low-fat milk every morning.

2. More protein, more calcium, plus fiber, vitamins, and minerals. By making a little extra and taking it to work, Joe manages to prepare two food opportunities in about 30 seconds. (Note: A little portable jug cooler keeps the smoothie's consistency—even if you put the blender glass in the fridge, the smoothie tends to separate after a few hours and become chalky.)

10 a.m. While he's still returning e-mail (ugh), he snacks on the almonds and fruit. That tides him over till lunchtime.[3]

Noon. If Joe can, he's off to the gym. (He avoids business lunches as much as possible; they suck time out of his day and suck control away from his diet.)

1 p.m. He'll usually grab a protein bar or protein shake at the gym.[4] Then he'll stroll over to the soup-and-sandwich joint, where he'll order a take-out spinach salad that's loaded with beans, corn, broccoli, red bell peppers, and tandoori chicken and topped with a half-ladle of balsamic vinegar.[5]

3 p.m. Joe's hungry (again). Fortunately, he's got a delicious smoothie hidden away in the office fridge. While others might be hitting their 3 p.m. slump, he's hitting the smoothie for a quick burst of energy.[6]

7:30 p.m. For the past 5 hours, Joe's been grinding away at work, so naturally he's ready for . . . more work. Joe has a business dinner almost every night. Dinner is his least disciplined part of the day, but the Abs Diet is pretty forgiving: His typical dinner starts with a chopped salad, then segues into beef ten-

3. More fiber and more vitamins, minerals, and protein. I can't stress enough the importance of stashing food in your office. Trail mix, dehydrated high-fiber soups and cereals, and fruit are staples of a workday diet. Once you stock your office with healthy snacks, you have seized control of your workday. When a meeting goes long and you can't get out for lunch, you've got healthy food on hand. Again, the more control you have over your food, the more you have over your body, and the more you have over your life.

4. More and more research indicates the importance of eating immediately after your workout, when your body is searching around for an energy source. If you eat immediately, your body uses the food to rebuild muscle; if you stay hungry, your body breaks down muscle for energy, and that's not good. I don't even like to wait the 10 minutes it takes between the gym and the take-out place; I eat immediately after my workout (though not in the locker room, which is just too gross).

5. More fiber, more protein, more vitamins and minerals. We're beginning to detect a pattern, Captain.

6. Yes, yes, we know . . . more protein, more calcium, more fiber. Does this guy ever stop?

derloin with a side of broccoli or green beans.[7] On top of that, he'll have some red wine and maybe a shared dessert.[8]

11 p.m. At home, Joe will often start grubbing around his refrigerator for something more to nosh on. He usually keeps a couple of cold cuts in there. Turkey, Swiss cheese, and a glass of fat-free milk will often complete his night.[9]

7. Order the steak; skip the mashed potatoes. A lot of us like to eat a lot at dinner, so at this meal, you simply keep carbs restricted as much as you can. That way, you can eat as much as you want.

8. Yes, it's okay to have dessert. Remember that high-fat, (high-sugar foods are for indulging, not for mindless snacking. Better to order the crème brûlée at a restaurant and really love it than mindlessly down half a bag of potato chips while watching TV—hundreds of fatty, salty calories that you won't remember eating 10 minutes later. Share the dessert with someone so that you get all the pleasure and half the guilt.

9. More calcium and more protein, including tryptophan, which is found in turkey and dairy products and helps induce sleep.

ABS DIET SUCCESS STORY

"I Solved My Back Pain— and Regained My Life!"

Name: Steve Toomey

Age: 39

Height: 6'3"

Starting weight: 215

Six weeks later: 195

When Steve Toomey would roll around in bed, he'd feel his back tense up at the slightest movement. It wasn't excruciating pain, but it was annoying—and it was interfering with his life.

"It really hampered my ability to play with my kids," he says. "I have one who's 6, one who's 5, one who's 3, and one on the way, and all they want to do is wrestle and roll around on the floor. All they were saying was, 'Daddy, when is your back going to get better so we can wrestle?'"

A doctor told him he needed to stretch his back. When he went back and said that stretching

How Stress Makes You Fat

ONE OF THE great side benefits of the Abs Diet is that it helps you take control of your life, which means taking control of your stress level. I can't emphasize strongly enough how important stress management is for your weight, for your health, and for the quality of life you'll lead.

That's because our bodies simply aren't designed to handle the stress of modern life. See, when stress hits, one of the first things your body does is jack up its production of adrenaline. Adrenaline causes fat cells all over your body to squirt their stores of fatty acids into your bloodstream to be used as energy. This was great back when stress meant a charging saber-toothed tiger or an attacking horde of barbarians and your fight-or-flight mechanism switched on. But it's not so great in today's society, where the only tigers and barbarians you have to handle are the ones who sign your paycheck. You don't flee or fight; you just bear down to get that report finished and munch your way through a midnight deadline. Meanwhile, your

wasn't helping, the doctor told him to give it one more chance and then they'd take an MRI. But that's when he started the Abs Diet.

"Once I incorporated the abs routine, the pain was gone," Toomey says. "Now I'm religious about the plan."

Since he started the program, he's lost 2 ½ inches from his waist, and he no longer has pain at night or fear that he's going to pull something when he's playing with the kids.

And in a house full of kids, where pizza and hot dogs are always on hand, Toomey has also appreciated the change in diet.

"The diet isn't nearly as restrictive as some of the diets I've tried, particularly the [ones with] super-low carbohydrates," he says. "On them, I used to crave slices of bread. Here, I can eat some carbs. I'm never starving or super hungry." But the biggest reward might be that weekly cheat meal. "My wife makes these Vietnamese egg rolls that are deep-fried, which I love. So I've been able to eat those on Sundays and not feel guilty," Toomey says. "I think that's really key—to be able to cheat once a week and know you're not going to ruin anything."

adrenal glands are producing yet another hormone to handle all that freshly released fat. It's called cortisol, but I want you to call it by its nickname: the belly-fat hormone.

In one Yale study, researchers asked 42 overweight people to perform an hour of stressful tasks—math problems, puzzles, and speech making. All the while, their cortisol levels were measured. The subjects who carried their extra weight in their bellies were discovered to be secreting more cortisol while under pressure. The theory runs like this: Stress hits, adrenaline mobilizes fat from all over the body, and cortisol takes the unused portion and stashes it with extreme prejudice toward the abdominal region. In a study of 438 male firefighters, the ones who said they worried about their financial security gained 11.2 pounds over 7 years, compared with an average of 7.4 pounds gained by nonworriers. The key to managing your midsection, then, is managing your stress. Here are a few proven ways to keep your head—and your abs—when all around you are losing theirs.

Skip Letterman. A University of Chicago study published in the journal *Sleep* showed that men who slept only 4 hours had cortisol levels 37 percent higher than men who got a full 8 hours of shut-eye; the men who stayed awake the whole night had levels 45 percent higher. Sleep specialists suggest that you strive for 8 hours per night.

Stop tossing and turning. How well you sleep matters, too. Another Uni-

|||||||||||||||||||||||||||||||||||||||||||||||||||||||||||||||||||||||||||||||||||||||||||||||||||||||||||||||||

Sneaky Ways to Keep Restaurants from Sabotaging Your Diet

▶ Many chefs pour at least an ounce of butter (200 calories and 23 grams of fat) onto a steak just so the meat will look juicier. Ask in advance and tell the cook to lay off.

▶ Those harmless-looking shredded carrots that dress up your beef are probably deep-fried; 1/2 cup is 137 calories (four times that of raw carrots) and 12 grams of fat. Skip 'em.

▶ If you go to a restaurant that serves salads tossed with dressing, it's usually a much lighter coating than what most people end up dumping on themselves, even if you order it on the side.

versity of Chicago study showed that men who got plenty of deep sleep—the quality stuff without all the dreaming and rapid eye movement—secreted almost 65 percent more human growth hormone (HGH) than men who were short on good slumber. You want more HGH to help prevent the loss of muscle mass caused by cortisol.

Remember C, as in "crisis." If you're in a stressful time of life—wondering why the jury has been out so long, perhaps—load up on vitamin C. For managing stress, you probably top out the benefit with a daily intake of 1,000 milligrams, divided into small doses throughout the day.

Don't have that last drink. Booze dehydrates you. Your body thinks there's a water shortage emergency, which bumps up your cortisol. How much alcohol is too much? Most of the smart money says three drinks a day. Same dehydration idea applies to caffeine. For cortisol control, stick to 200 milligrams per day, about what you get in two cups of coffee.

Take the wheel. A sense of control over some of the stressors in your life helps. "If you blast a volunteer randomly with a noise, his stress hormones rise," says Robert Sapolsky, PhD, professor of biological and neurological sciences at Stanford University. "But if you give him a button and tell him that pressing it will decrease the likelihood of the noise, there's a smaller stress response to the same sound." Getting organized, even in small ways, may help you feel more like the captain of your ship.

Make a plan. "People manage stress more effectively if they can believe that things are improving," says Sapolsky. So make sure you always have something you're looking forward to. Hope makes stress manageable.

Get spiritual. Remember the simple wisdom of Simone Weil: Any undivided attention is prayer. If we can stop the tumble in our heads and every day briefly commit our complete attention to something—a 10-foot putt, a 10-penny nail, or a 10-year-old child—we may acquire the serenity many find in formal faith.

Chapter 11

TURBOCHARGING THE NEW ABS DIET

How Exercise Can Strip Away Fat and Add Muscle

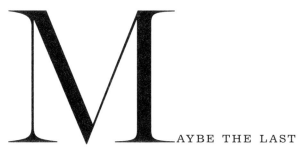

AYBE THE LAST few months, years, or decades of your life have been one big snowstorm— a snowstorm of office parties and happy hours, of vending machine dinners, of midnight pizza deliveries. When you're a kid, those storms can be fun, but as you get older, they're more of a mess than anything else. They dump pounds and pounds of fat onto your once-svelte gut, leaving your abs buried deep under everything. No sun's going to melt your fat after a couple of days, and no snowblower's going to suck it up and shoot it over to the neighbor's lawn. (But how cool would that be?)

If you want to see the sidewalk, you have to shovel the snow. If you want to find your abs, you have to burn the fat.

Eating right is critical, and yes, by following the nutrition principles of the New Abs Diet and centering your meals around the Abs Diet Powerfoods, you'll lose fat pretty effortlessly. But to maximize your weight loss and turn your fat into muscle, this book includes something other diet books ignore: a quick-and-easy exercise plan. Exercise will not only make you healthier; it'll make you lose weight faster. It'll make you stronger. Most important, it'll make your body turn fat into muscle—by converting energy that's stored in fat into energy that feeds muscle.

The New Abs Diet Workout Principles

HAVING WORKED AT *Men's Health* for more than 17 years, I know all the latest trends in exercise, but I also scour the latest and most credible scientific research measuring the effectiveness of various workout plans. With that knowledge, I've constructed the exercise portion of the plan to help you burn fat at the highest levels possible in the least amount of time. I know you don't have time to spend hours a day exercising, so I want you to get the most out of every workout. And I know that flexibility and convenience are the keys to formulating a plan you can stick to, so I've created a workout you can do in your local gym—or in your living room. This plan allows you to keep your workouts short and focused, while still keeping you on target for your ultimate goal. Pound for pound, it's the best workout possible for finding your abs. These are the workout principles.

Focus on your diet first. The first 2 weeks of exercise are optional. If you already exercise regularly, you can jump right into the New Abs Diet Workout, and you should, because you'll burn even more fat than with the New Abs Diet alone. But if you're a beginner or you haven't exercised in a long time, take the first 2 weeks to adjust to your new eating plan before starting the workout.

ABS DIET SUCCESS STORY

"I Regained My Self-Esteem!"

Name: Brian Archiquette

Age: 35

Height: 6'3"

Starting weight: 275

Six weeks later: 250

After reaching his all-time high of 345 pounds, Brian Archiquette signed up for the gym. He had steadily gained 130 pounds after getting married 9 years ago, and he had finally had it. He was tired of being fat. He felt miserable and depressed. "I felt like I was standing on the sidelines of life," he says.

Add in the fact that his father died of congestive heart failure and that he was headed in the same direction, and Archiquette knew he had to make a change—and he'd have to do it now. He followed workouts in

If you're champing at the bit to begin maximizing your weight loss, start getting in the exercise habit by walking briskly for up to 30 minutes a day.

Focus on muscles. I used to work with a guy who was about 30 pounds overweight. He decided he'd enter a race as motivation to help him lose weight. He ran 6 days a week and followed his running program religiously, but he didn't lose a pound. Sure, he was able to run farther than he ever had, but his body stayed the same. Why? First, because he still based his diet around pizza, pasta, and wings, and second, because steady-state cardiovascular exercise doesn't burn fat the way strength training does. (Incidentally, when the same guy went on the Abs Diet and started a weight-lifting program, he lost nearly 20 pounds in less than 2 months.)

Your muscles are hungry little suckers, and in order to keep themselves well nourished, they want to burn those calories you're eating. So the more muscle you have, the more calories you eliminate—in the gym, at work, even in bed. This program focuses on working your large muscle groups—legs, chest, back, and shoulders—because that's where you can build the most muscle in the least amount of time. Plus, when you work your larger muscles, you fire up your metabolism by creating a longer calorie afterburn—lasting right up to your next workout!

Men's Health magazine and gradually dropped to 275 pounds. When he went on the Abs Diet, he supercharged the weight loss and dropped an additional 25 pounds in 6 weeks.

"It was planning the meals and the timing of the meals. I was trying to balance the meals throughout the day, plus add the exercise," says Archiquette, whose weakness is pizza. "In the past, what would happen is that I wouldn't eat, and then I'd overeat because I got so hungry."

While he's on his way to reaching his goal of weighing 215 pounds on his 6-foot-3 frame, he's already made tremendous gains. He's dropped from a 48-inch waist to a 40-inch waist. And now when he walks through the mall, he doesn't have to find a place to sit down every couple of minutes. The biggest gain, he says, has been in his self-esteem.

"I definitely have more energy and a more positive outlook on life," he says. "I'm more confident—even when I'm standing in front of people at work. I was always self-conscious, thinking that they're looking at my belly sticking out or that my shirt is too tight. Now I feel better about myself."

Think about the small fraction of time you spend exercising. Even if you work out four or five times a day for an hour at a time, that's nothing compared to the amount of time you're not exercising every day. So in order to gain the most metabolic benefit, you want to maximize the calories you're burning when you're not working out.

Focus on spending less time in the gym. The New Abs Diet Workout employs two simple concepts to maximize muscle growth and fat-burning and minimize the time you spend exercising.

Circuit training. This term refers to performing different exercises one right after another. For example, we'll have you do a set of leg exercises followed immediately by a set of an upper-body exercise, until you do 8 to 10 different exercises in a row. There are two reasons circuit training works. First, by cutting down the rest periods between exercises, circuit training keeps your heart rate elevated throughout your training session, maximizing your fat burn while providing tremendous cardiovascular fitness benefits. Second, circuit training keeps your workout short—you won't waste time resting between sets of an exercise, which means you can get on with the rest of your busy life.

Compound exercises. Another key part of the strength-training program is compound exercises, that is, exercises that call into play multiple muscle

||||||||||||||||||||||||||||||||||||||||||||||||||||||||||||||||||||||||||||||||||||||||||||||||||||||||||||

Abs Facts

Stay slow and steady. Here's a trick: Slowly say the phrase "slow and controlled" to yourself as you curl your body upward during an abdominal crunch. It should take at least as much time to reach the top of the movement as it does to say this mantra (same goes for the way down).

Stretch it out. If your hamstrings are tight, you may develop a habit of leaning backward to relieve the pressure. This posture tends to thrust your gut forward, making your paunch look even paunchier. Stretching your hamstrings a few times a week should help. If you're already stretched—for time, that is—the fastest, easiest way to loosen up your back and hamstrings and tighten your abdomen is by doing what's called the Figure-4 Stretch. Here's how to do it: Sit on the floor with your right leg straight in front of you, toes pointing up. Bend your left knee to place your left heel against the inside of your right thigh, near your groin; keep your left knee almost touching the floor. Now reach out slowly with your right arm and touch your right toe. If you can't do it, try grabbing your ankle. Hold the

groups rather than just focusing on one. For example, with the New Abs Diet Workout, we don't want you to exercise your chest, and then your shoulders, and then your triceps, and then your forearms. We want you to hit many different muscles at the same time and then get out of the gym. One study showed that you can put on 6 pounds of muscle and lose 15 pounds of fat in 6 weeks by following an exercise program that employs the compound exercises found in the New Abs Diet Workout. What's even better is that those subjects followed an exercise plan for only 20 minutes three times a week. Not only do compound exercises make your workout more fun and more challenging, they will also increase the demands on your muscles—even though you're not actually doing more work. (For instance, the squat hits a whopping 256 muscles with just one movement!) Greater muscle demand triggers your body to produce more human growth hormone—a potent fat burner.

By working more muscle, your body uses more energy to repair and upgrade it the day after your workout. A 2008 study at Syracuse University showed that people burned more calories the day after they performed lower-body resistance training exercises than the day after they worked their upper bodies simply because the leg muscles generally have more mass than the muscles in the chest and arms.

||||||||||||||||||||||||||||||||||||||||||||||||||||||||||||||||||||||||||||||||||||||||||||||||||||||||||||

position for 30 seconds, return to the starting position, and then stretch again for another 30 seconds. Switch legs, and stretch your left side twice also.

Kick the butts. Research shows that smokers have a greater abdomen-to-hip ratio than former smokers or people who never smoked. That means smokers are more likely to put on pounds around their midsections. It's yet another reason to put down those cancer sticks for good.

Think small. Sure, excess calories lead to excess weight. But how and when you eat are just as important as what. Eating large meals, for example, can actually stretch your abdominal muscles outward. Stuff yourself on a regular basis, and your abs will become so stretched that they'll lose their ability to rein in your gut. That's another reason why multiple small meals are better than a few large ones.

Get some flex time. When you're sitting in your car or at your desk, tense your middle as you would at the start of the crunch. Sit up straight and pull your abs in for 60 seconds at a time, at least once an hour. Anytime you feel them going slack throughout your day, tighten them up again.

If the only weight you've ever picked up is around your gut and not in the gym, don't worry that you're not familiar with working with weights. You can start by lifting any amount of weight that you're comfortable with—whether it's a pair of light dumbbells or a couple of cans of beans. Even if you start small, you'll grow stronger, start to build muscle, and keep your metabolism revved. As you progress, you'll build and burn more.

Focus on intensity. Go back to the guy I worked with. He ran 6 days a week, but he ran as slow as the ketchup at the bottom of the bottle. His intensity never

||||||||||||||||||||||||||||||||||||||||||||||||||||||||||||||||||||||||||||||||||||||||||||||||||||||||||

Workout Struggles

We all have times when it's tough to psych ourselves up for our workout routines. Here's a rundown of the most common workout obstacles and the best ways to get past them.

Strength training: So what if it's 8 reps or 12? Whether you're doing crunches, bench presses, or lunges, it's easy to lose motivation when you're doing rep after rep after rep.
The Fix: Keep your eye on your goals. You build strength when your muscles break down and your body repairs them by creating tougher muscle tissue. You barely begin to break down muscles during the first few reps, which is why you need to pick a weight that allows you to complete 10 challenging yet doable reps without compromising form.

Running: Sore legs. If your body is producing lactic acid during one of the interval sessions that you'll learn about on page 206, it can cause a burning sensation in your quads and glutes. That soreness is pain you can push through and a positive indicator of how hard you're working.
The Fix: Resting for a minute or two will allow your body to take in more oxygen, which you need to help flush the lactic acid. Stretch while you rest to separate the muscle fibers and improve circulation. Try the Stork to stretch quads and hips: Stand on one leg and pull the other behind you, bringing your heel toward your butt.

Cardio machines: Boring! Your brain is zoning out, and your body needs new stimulation as it adapts to repetitive movement patterns.
The Fix: All the more reason to make your cardio workouts interval sessions. They'll trick your mind into thinking the workout is moving quicker. Plus, you'll challenge your muscles, burning more calories and building strength. Do 2 minutes at a fast pace, then drop it down for 1 minute, alternating until you're out of time. (See "How to Improve Your Cardio Machine Workouts," page 207.)

---

elevated, and because of that, he never burned that much fat. Time and time again, research has shown that higher-intensity workouts promote weight loss better than steady-state activities. In a Canadian study from Laval University, researchers measured differences in fat loss between two groups of exercisers following two different workout programs. The first group rode stationary bikes four or five times a week and burned 300 to 400 calories per 30- to 45-minute session. The second group did the same, but only one or two times a week, and they filled the rest of their sessions with short intervals of high-intensity cycling. They hopped on their stationary bikes and pedaled as quickly as they could for 30 to 90 seconds, rested, and then repeated the process several times per exercise session. As a result, they burned 225 to 250 calories while cycling, but they had burned more fat at the end of the study than the workers in the first group. In fact, even though they exercised less, their fat loss was nine times greater. Researchers said that the majority of the fat burning took place after the workout.

The New Abs Diet Workout recommends that you add one simple interval workout per week to complement your strength training. These are workouts of traditional cardiovascular exercise (running, swimming, biking) in which you alternate between periods of high intensity and periods of rest. (I'll explain more about how to create an effective interval workout in the next chapter.)

If You Don't Already Exercise

THE BEST PART about the 6-week New Abs Diet Workout is that, for the first 2 weeks at least, you don't actually have to exercise. If you're not doing anything in the way of a workout right now, it's not critical that you start the program immediately. Instead, I want you to concentrate on acclimating your body and your schedule to the New Abs Diet. Take it slow at first.

If You're Already in the Exercise Habit

MAYBE YOU LIFT weights once or twice a week. Maybe you jog a few miles every morning. Maybe you're favored to win the gold in the decathlon this summer. I dunno. What I do know is that no matter what your workout is now, you're probably going to build more muscle, and burn more fat, if you switch to the New Abs Diet Workout.

Even if your current exercise program has been working well for you, experts agree that mixing up your workout every month or so is the best way to maximize your results. That's because gains in strength and overall fitness come from challenging your body to perform in ways it's not used to. Performing the same workout over and over again doesn't train your body to reach its potential; it just trains your body to be really, really good at performing that one workout. So I want you to consider switching your current workout over to the New Abs Diet Workout, at least for a few weeks. I guarantee the results you'll see will be astounding.

The New Abs Diet Workout: Suggested Weekly Schedule

YOU CAN MIX and match the different workouts to meet your lifestyle needs. When you construct your schedule, make sure to:

▶ Leave at least 48 hours between weight workouts of the same body parts. Your muscles need time to recover and repair themselves after a workout.

|||||||||||||||||||||||||||||||||||||||||||||||||||||||||||||||||||||||||||||||||||||||||||||||||||||||

Quick Tips for Lean Abs

Move faster: Target your fast-twitch muscle fibers and you'll build stronger abs in less time. Spanish researchers found that doing abdominal exercises at a fast tempo activates more muscle than doing them slowly. Crank out as many reps as you can do in 20 seconds for a more effective core workout in less time.

Focus on the flip side: Your abs are an intricate system of muscles, connecting to your rib cage, your hips, and even your backbone. To have strong abs, you need not only belly exercises but also lower-back strength and exercises for your obliques (the abdominal muscles that run down the sides of your torso). All these core muscles work together. By strengthening them, you'll not only improve the look of your abs, but you'll protect yourself from throwing out your back.

Don't sacrifice your best ally: When you lose weight on a typical "diet," muscle is the first thing to go. It's more expensive for your body to retain than fat is, so when you run low on calories, your body dumps muscle mass and turns it into energy. (That's why diets of denial are counterproductive.) When you go off diets of sacrifice, you begin to gain back the pounds—but because

▶ Take 1 day each week to rest with no formal exercise.

▶ Warm up for 5 minutes before starting to exercise, either through a light jog, riding on a stationary bike, jumping rope, or doing slow jumping jacks.

The three components of your weekly schedule include:

1. Strength training: Three times a week. These are total-body workouts with one workout that puts extra emphasis on your legs.

2. Additional cardiovascular exercise: Optional, on non-strength-training days. Examples are cycling, running, swimming, walking, and using cardio machines. An interval workout is recommended for 1 day a week, and light cardiovascular exercise like walking is recommended for 2 of your 3 off days.

3. Abs exercises: Twice a week. I recommend doing them before your strength training or interval workouts; you'll be less likely to skip them (more on abs exercises in Chapter 13).

||||||||||||||||||||||||||||||||||||||||||||||||||||||||||||||||||||||||||||||||||||||||||||||||||||||||||||||||||||||||||||||||||||||||||||||||

you now have less calorie-burning muscle on your frame, the weight you gain is fat. By dieting, you've effectively turned muscle into fat.

Exercise, then eat: Research suggests that the best way to eat less at a meal is to work out right before it. This works in several ways: First, you're less hungry when your metabolism is revving, such as right after a workout. Second, you're thirstier, so you drink more water, which uses up space in your belly and relieves hunger. Third, the calories you do eat get burned for energy pronto—not stored as fat.

Stand taller: When you're walking, stand tall and picture a cape flowing off your shoulders, Superman-style, to ensure your best posture. A taller posture will give you the appearance of being slimmer, while also training your abs to stay taut.

Practice looking leaner: Maybe you've heard of "muscle memory": the way your body learns to do a physical activity (like riding a bike) and never forgets. Well, your abs have a memory, too. If you consciously keep your abs firm throughout the day, they'll tend to stay firm even when you're relaxed.

Chapter 12

THE NEW ABS DIET WORKOUT

The Easiest, Most Effective Workout Plan Ever

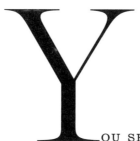

OU SEE EVERY KIND OF person in the gym. The guy with no fat. The guy with no neck. The guy with lots of fat. The guy with lots of necks. And it seems they all get there a different way. I know that guys have as many different workout philosophies as they have pirated MP3 files, but the one guy I really know I can help is the overweight man who's working his forearm muscles by doing wrist curls in the corner. He's like a guy who has totaled his car but wants to get the radio fixed first. There's no point working on the fine points until you've taken care of the bigger issues.

That's why I've built a total-body strength training workout: to increase your lean muscle mass as efficiently as possible. It's simple: To show off your abs, you have to burn fat. To burn fat, you have to build muscle. Remember that adding just 1 pound of muscle will force your body to burn up to an additional 50 calories a day, every day.

This workout emphasizes the larger muscle groups of your body—chest, back, and legs. In one workout during the week, you'll give extra attention to your legs. I know what you're thinking: My abs are up here. Why do I care about working what's down there? Because most of your body's muscle is found below your belly button. Your lower body is where you'll build the most muscle in the least amount of time; working this giant muscle mass triggers the release of large amounts of growth hormone, which in turn stimulates muscle growth throughout your body, kicks your fat burners into overdrive, and gives you that washboard stomach you want—in no time flat. Indeed, leg exercises are the key to total-body strength: In one Norwegian study, men who focused on lower-body work gained more upper-body strength than did those who emphasized upper-body exercises in their workouts. That doesn't mean you'll ignore your upper body entirely, though. With the upper-body workout, you'll also work your largest muscles—your chest, back, and shoulders—to burn more fat. If you follow this program, you'll still notice more growth and definition in your whole body—even your forearms, even your shoulders, and, yes, even your abs—and you'll begin to reshape your body.

Here, you're going to do circuit training to optimize your muscle-building potential. That is, you'll perform one set of an exercise and then move immediately to the next exercise, with just 30 seconds of rest. Follow the order of the exercises I've listed on the following pages; that will allow you to work different body parts from set to set. (A complete set of exercise descriptions and instructional photos begins on page 184.) By alternating between body parts, you'll keep your body in constant work mode and be able to perform the movements back-to-back without rest. Here's why circuit training works so well: You'll save time because you'll cut the amount of rest you need when you alternate muscle groups. More important, you'll keep your heart rate elevated throughout the workout, so you'll burn even more fat while you're exercising— whether it's in the gym or in your own living room.

In the first 2 weeks of the program, do the circuit twice. Move from exercise to exercise with no more than 30 seconds of rest in between. When you complete one circuit, rest for 1 to 2 minutes, then complete the second circuit. After the first 2 weeks, when you've become comfortable doing two complete circuits during a workout, increase your workload to three circuits per workout. In every exercise, use a weight that you can handle comfortably for the number of repetitions noted. When that becomes too easy, increase the weight on each set by 10 percent or less. Here's a sample schedule of how you might arrange your workouts.

MONDAY:
Total-Body Strength Training Workout with Ab Emphasis
Complete one set of each ab exercise*, then complete the rest of the circuit twice.

EXERCISE	REPETITIONS	REST	SETS
Traditional Crunch*	12–15	none	1
Bent-Leg Knee Raise*	12–15	none	1
Oblique V-Up*	10 each side	none	1
Bridge*	1 or 2	none	1
Back Extension*	12–15	none	1
Squat	10–12	30 seconds	2
Bench Press	10	30 seconds	2
Pulldown	10	30 seconds	2
Military Press	10	30 seconds	2
Upright Row	10	30 seconds	2
Triceps Pushdown	10–12	30 seconds	2
Leg Extension	10–12	30 seconds	2
Biceps Curl	10	30 seconds	2
Leg Curl	10–12	30 seconds	2

TUESDAY (OPTIONAL):
Light Cardiovascular Exercise Such as Walking
Try for 30 minutes at a brisk pace.

WEDNESDAY:
Total-Body Strength Training Workout with Ab Emphasis
Complete one set of each ab exercise*, then complete the rest of the circuit twice.

EXERCISE	REPETITIONS	REST	SETS
Standing Crunch*	12–15	none	1
Pulse-Up*	12	none	1
Saxon Side Bend*	6–10 each side	none	1

(chart continued)

Side Bridge*	1 or 2 each side	none	1
Back Extension*	12–15	none	1
Squat	10–12	30 seconds	2
Bench Press	10	30 seconds	2
Pulldown	10	30 seconds	2
Military Press	10	30 seconds	2
Upright Row	10	30 seconds	2
Triceps Pushdown	10–12	30 seconds	2
Leg Extension	10–12	30 seconds	2
Biceps Curl	10	30 seconds	2
Leg Curl	10–12	30 seconds	2

THURSDAY (OPTIONAL):
Light Cardiovascular Exercise Such as Walking
Try for 30–45 minutes at a brisk pace.

FRIDAY:
Total-Body Strength Training Workout with Leg Emphasis
Repeat entire circuit twice.

EXERCISE	REPETITIONS	REST	SETS
Squat	10–12	30 seconds	2
Bench Press	10	30 seconds	2
Pulldown	10	30 seconds	2
Traveling Lunge	10–12 each leg	30 seconds	2
Military Press	10	30 seconds	2
Upright Row	10	30 seconds	2
Step-Up	10–12 each leg	30 seconds	2
Triceps Pushdown	10–12	30 seconds	2
Leg Extension	10–12	30 seconds	2
Biceps Curl	10	30 seconds	2
Leg Curl	10–12	30 seconds	2

SATURDAY (OPTIONAL):
Abs Workout Plus Interval Workout
Complete one set of each ab exercise, then choose one interval workout from the selection on pages 206 and 209.

EXERCISE	REPETITIONS	REST	SETS
Traditional Crunch	12–15	none	1
Bent-Leg Knee Raise	12	none	1
Oblique V-Up	6–10 each side	none	1
Bridge	1 or 2	none	1
Back Extension	12–15	none	1

SUNDAY: OFF

||||||||||||||||||||||||||||||||||||||||||||||||||||||||||||||||||||||||||||||||||||||||||||||||||||||||||||||||||||||||

Dumbbell Smarts

When it comes to versatility, ease of use, and pure effectiveness, no muscle-building equipment beats dumbbells. On a practical level, they're inexpensive, indestructible, and compact. (Just try stuffing a Soloflex under the bed!) Eight reasons why smart folks surround themselves with dumbbells:

1. Dumbbells give you a more complete workout. You may think of dumbbells only in terms of biceps curls, but they're effective for working your legs (lunges, calf raises), back (deadlifts), and abdominals (side bends, weighted crunches) as well.

2. Dumbbells challenge your muscles more. When your body becomes used to a given workout, it stops being challenged, and your muscles stop growing. Because there are hundreds of different exercises you can do with dumbbells, you can keep updating your workout, so your muscles stay challenged—and keep growing.

3. Dumbbells build greater strength. Because they allow for a greater range of motion during exercise, dumbbells challenge your muscles in ways no other equipment can. For example, a barbell becomes restricting during a bench press because you can bring the weight down only so far before your chest gets in the way. But when you're holding a dumbbell in each hand, you can bring the weight down lower during each repetition, calling into play more muscle fiber and stimulating more growth.

4. Dumbbells build strength faster. Negative resistance training refers to the stress you put on your muscles during the lowering, or negative, phase of an exercise. And negative resistance may grow muscle even more effectively than the positive, or lifting, phase of an exercise. With dumbbells, you can add extra negative resistance into your workout. Let's say you've done 10 biceps curls with your left hand, and you can't possibly lift the weight one more time. You can now use your right hand to help your left lift the weight one more time, and simply lower the dumbbell using your left hand only. This helps you squeeze out that last little bit of benefit from your workout.

5. Dumbbells can give you a healthier heart. Plenty of studies have shown that weight training reduces blood pressure and indirectly strengthens the heart. Researchers have also shown that a dumbbell workout can yield additional benefits, including a lower lipid profile (less gum for your arteries) and increased oxygen uptake. Dumbbells do a better job at this than other weight training, again because of the greater range of motion they allow.

6. Dumbbells make you work in three dimensions: They don't lock you into the up-and-down or side-to-side motions that exercise machines do. That means your muscles learn to function well in real life, whether you're catching the winning pass in the neighborhood game or catching the kids before they fall off the swings.

||||||||||||||||||||||||||||||||||||||||||||||||||||||||||||||||||||||||||||||||||||||||||||||||||||

7. Dumbbells keep your body in balance. By forcing each arm to lift its fair share, dumbbells help to immediately identify strength imbalances that may have developed from sports, from simple acts like driving or carrying a briefcase, or from lifting with barbells or machines. When pressing a barbell overhead, for example, you can compensate for a weaker left arm by pushing more with your right side—and just make the imbalance worse. When you're pressing two dumbbells overhead, however, each side of your body has to work independently—and each side gets the same amount of exercise.

8. Dumbbells help prevent injury. While exercise machines are calibrated to target one muscle exclusively, dumbbles strengthen you everywhere, especially in the important but often overlooked small muscles, ligaments, and tendons. Machines may miss these, setting you up for injury.

THE 10-MINUTE TOTAL-BODY DUMBBELL PUMP

When you don't have time for a longer workout, try this super-fast dumbbell combination lift. It works every major muscle group in one speedy circuit. Do two to three sets of 10 repetitions, and you're done for the day.

Warmup: Start by doing 5 minutes of calesthenics (jumping jacks, bodyweight squats, rope jumping, whatever you wish) to warm up your muscles.

Step 1: Grab a pair of lightweight dumbbells and get into a pushup position, with your arms straight and directly beneath your shoulders and your hands on the dumbbells. Use hexagonal dumbbells, so they won't roll when you do the pushup.

Step 2: Do a pushup. Then bring your feet underneath you, one foot at a time.

Step 3: Keeping your back flat, stand up. (This is a deadlift.)

Step 4: From the standing position, curl the weights up to your shoulders.

Step 5: Swing your elbows out to your sides so that the weights are above your shoulders. Lower your body until your thighs are parallel to the floor. Pause, then stand up as you press the weights overhead. (This combines a weighted squat with an overhead press.)

Step 6: Lower the weights to your sides. Bend your knees, place the dumbbells on the floor shoulder-width apart and get back into pushup position with your hands on the dumbbells. Now repeat the steps for a total of 10 repetitions.

Basic Exercises

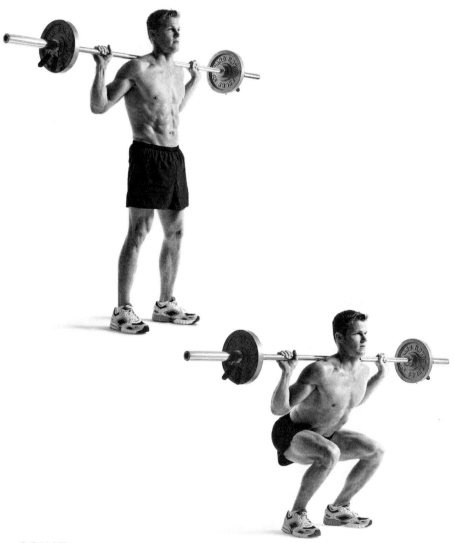

SQUAT

Hold a barbell with an overhand grip so that it rests comfortably on your upper back. Set your feet shoulder-width apart, and keep your knees slightly bent, back straight, and eyes focused straight ahead. Slowly lower your body as if you were sitting back into a chair, keeping your back in its natural alignment and your lower legs nearly perpendicular to the floor. When your thighs are parallel to the floor, pause, then return to the starting position.

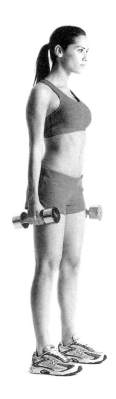

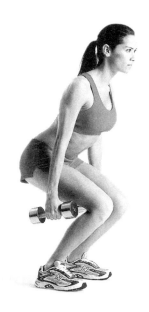

HOME VARIATION: *Same, but with one dumbbell in each hand, your palms facing your outer thighs.*

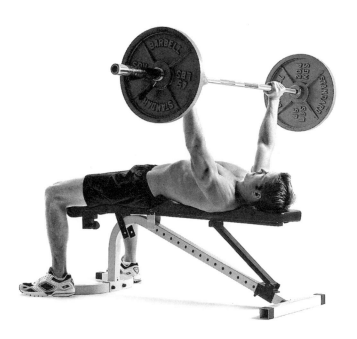

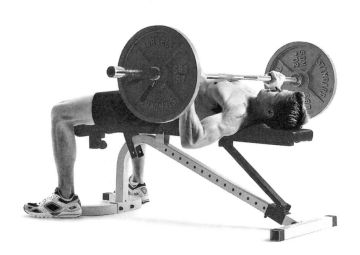

BENCH PRESS

Lie on your back on a flat bench with your feet on the floor. Grab the barbell with an overhand grip, your hands just beyond shoulder-width apart. Lift the bar off the uprights, and hold it at arm's length over your chest. Slowly lower the bar to your chest. Pause, then push the bar back to the starting position.

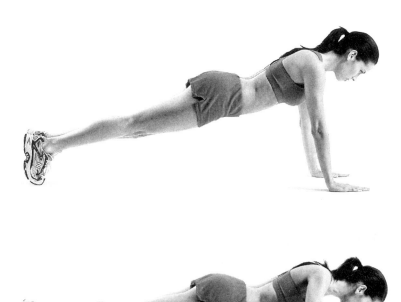

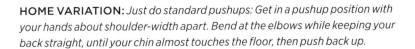

HOME VARIATION: *Just do standard pushups: Get in a pushup position with your hands about shoulder-width apart. Bend at the elbows while keeping your back straight, until your chin almost touches the floor, then push back up.*

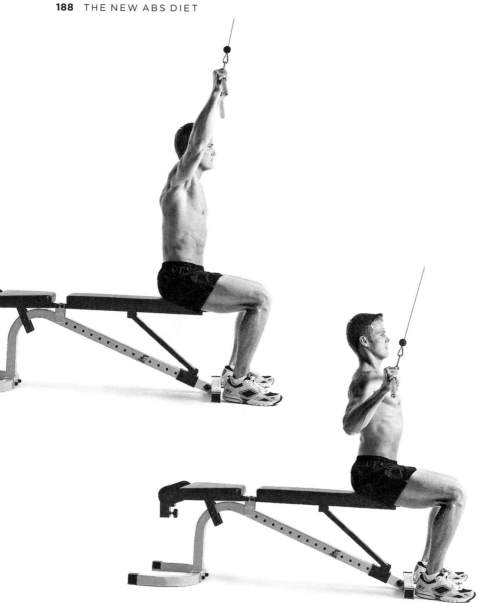

PULLDOWN

Stand facing a lat pulldown machine. Reach up and grasp the bar with an over-hand grip that's 4 to 6 inches wider than your shoulders. Sit on the seat, letting the resistance of the bar extend your arms above your head. When you're in position, pull the bar down until it touches your upper chest. Hold this position for a second, then return to the starting position.

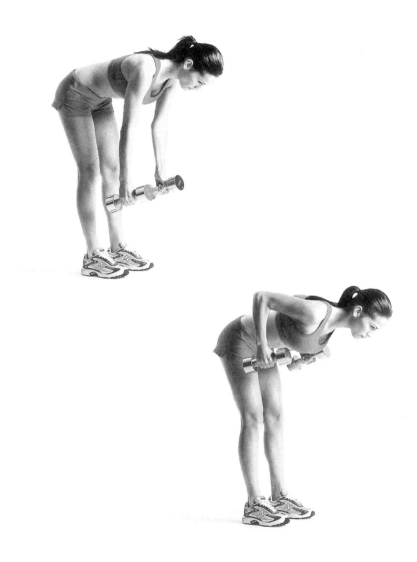

HOME VARIATION: *Bent-over row. Stand with your knees slightly bent and shoulder-width apart. Bend over so that your back is almost parallel to the floor. Holding a dumbbell in each hand, let your arms hang toward the floor. With your palms facing in, pull the dumbbells toward you until they touch the outside of your chest. Pause, then return to the starting position.*

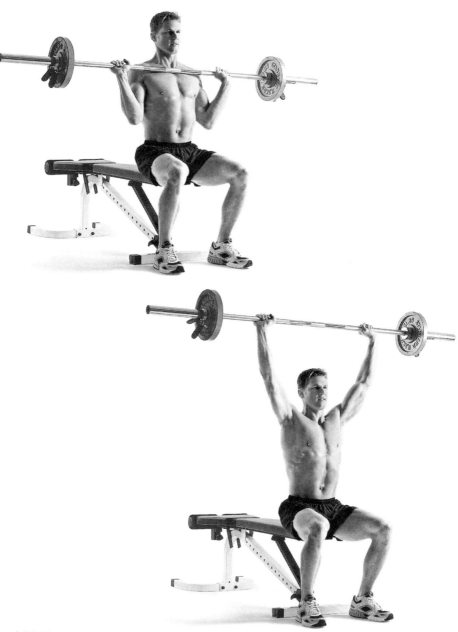

MILITARY PRESS

Sitting on an exercise bench, hold a barbell at shoulder height with your hands shoulder-width apart. Press the weight straight overhead so that your arms are almost fully extended, hold for a count of one, then bring it down to the front of your shoulders. Repeat.

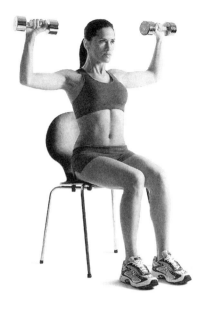

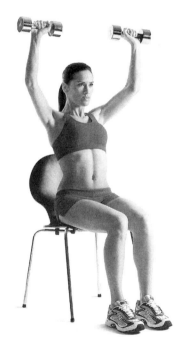

HOME VARIATION: *Sitting on a sturdy chair instead of a bench, hold one dumb-bell in each hand, about level with your ears. Push the dumbbells straight overhead so that your arms are almost fully extended, hold for a count of one, then return to the starting position. Repeat.*

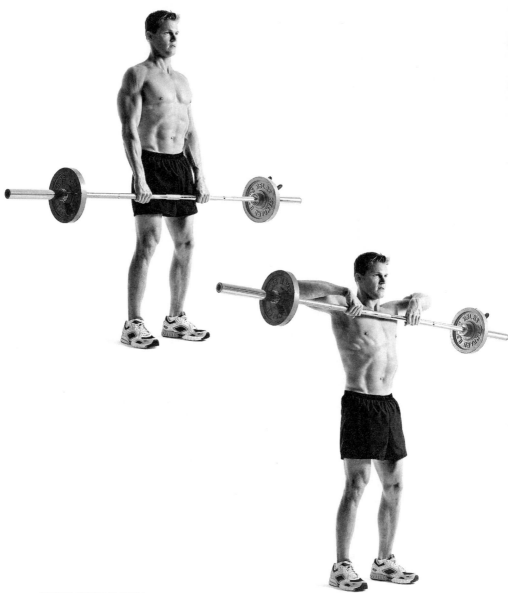

UPRIGHT ROW

Grab a barbell with an overhand grip, and stand with your feet shoulder-width apart and your knees slightly bent. Let the barbell hang at arm's length on top of your thighs, thumbs pointed toward each other. Bending your elbows, lift your upper arms straight out to the sides, and pull the barbell straight up until your upper arms are parallel to the floor and the bar is just below chin level. Pause, then return to the starting position.

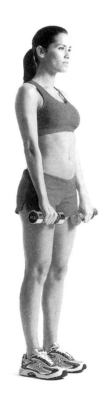

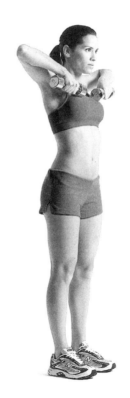

HOME VARIATION: *Same, using one dumbbell in each hand.*

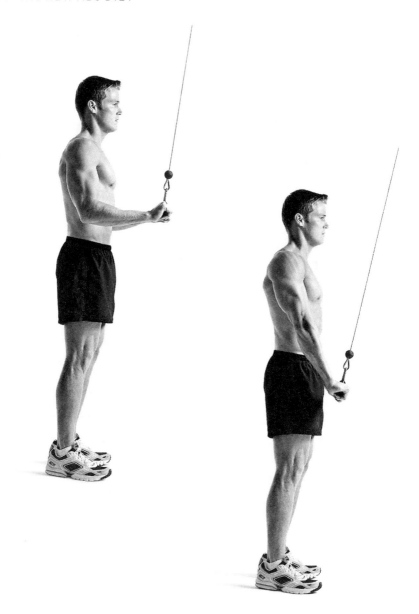

TRICEPS PUSHDOWN

While standing, grip a bar attached to a high pulley cable or lat machine with your hands about 6 inches apart. With your elbows tucked against your sides, bring the bar down until it is directly in front of you. With your forearms parallel to the floor (the starting position), push the bar down until your arms are extended straight down with the bar near your thighs. Don't lock your elbows. Return to the starting position.

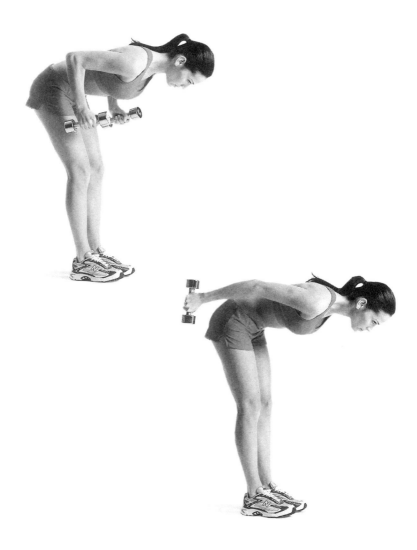

HOME VARIATION: *Triceps kickback. Stand with your knees slightly bent and shoulder-width apart. Bend over so that your back is almost parallel to the ground. Bend your elbows to about 90-degree angles, raising them to just above the level of your back. This is the starting position. Extend your forearms backward, keeping your upper arms stationary. When they're fully extended, your arms should be parallel to the ground. Pause, then return to the starting position.*

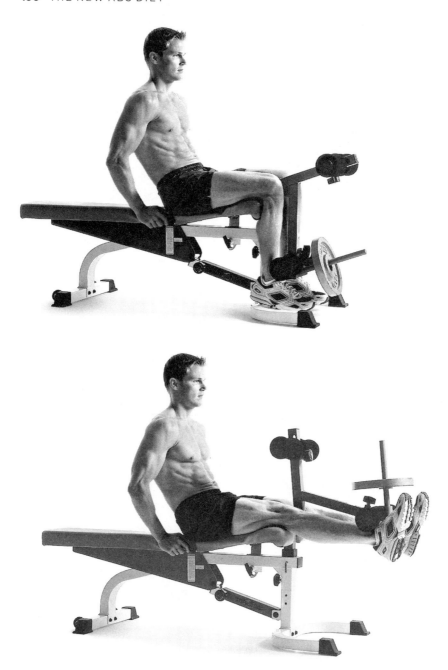

LEG EXTENSION

Sitting on a leg extension machine with your feet under the footpads, lean back slightly, and lift the pads with your feet until your legs are extended.

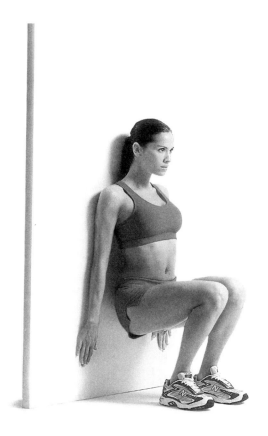

HOME VARIATION: *Squat against the wall. Stand with your back flat against a wall. Squat down so that your thighs are parallel to the ground. Hold that position for as long as you can. That consists of one set. Aim for 20 seconds to start, and work your way up to 45 seconds.*

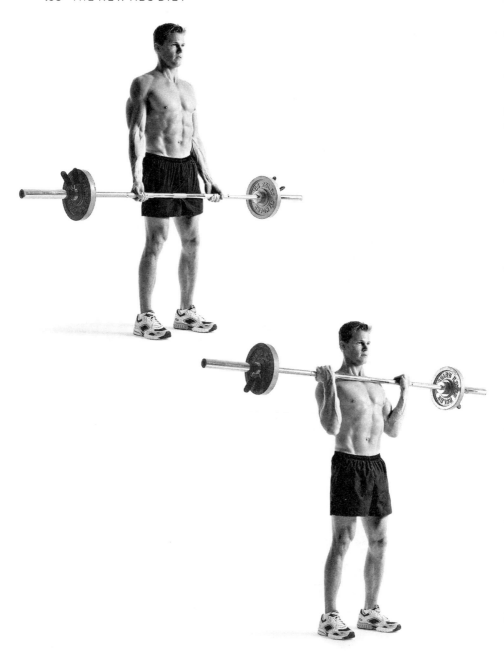

BICEPS CURL

Stand while holding a barbell in front of you, palms facing out, with your hands shoulder-width apart and your arms hanging in front of you. Curl the weight toward your shoulders, hold for a second, then return to the starting position.

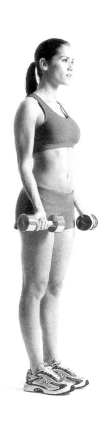

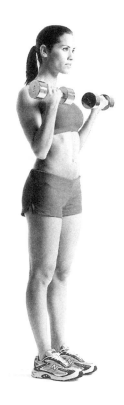

HOME VARIATION: *Same, only use a set of dumbbells instead.*

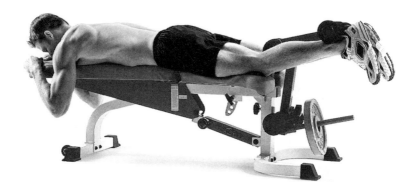

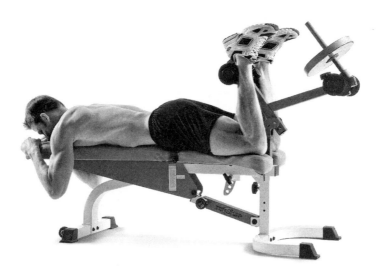

LEG CURL

Lie facedown on a leg curl machine, and hook your ankles under the padded bar. Keeping your stomach and pelvis against the bench, slowly raise your feet toward your butt, curling up the weight. Come up so that your feet nearly touch your butt, and slowly return to the starting position.

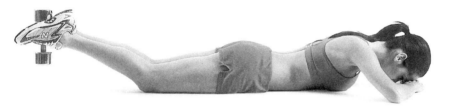

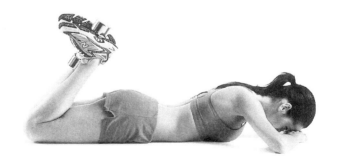

HOME VARIATION: *Lie down with your stomach on the floor. Put a light dumb-bell between your feet (so that the top end of the dumbbell rests on the bottom of your feet). Squeeze your feet together, and curl them up toward your butt.*

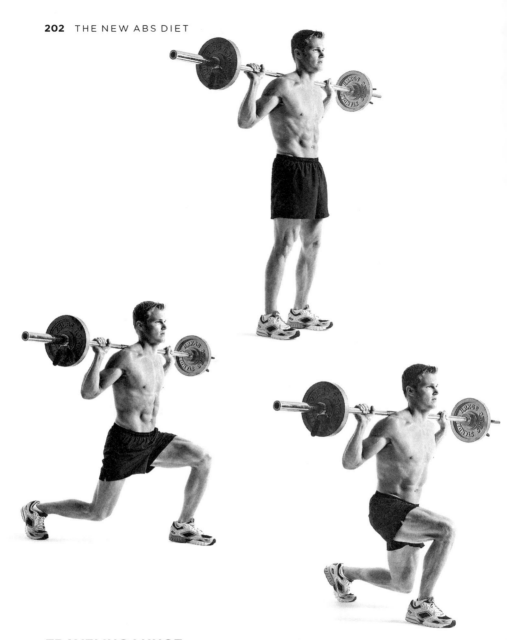

TRAVELING LUNGE

Rest a barbell across your upper back. Stand, with your feet hip-width apart, at one end of the room; you need room to walk about 20 steps. Step forward with your left foot, and lower your body so that your left thigh is parallel to the floor and your right thigh is perpendicular to the floor (your right knee should bend and almost touch the floor). Stand and bring your right foot up next to your left, then repeat with the right leg lunging forward.

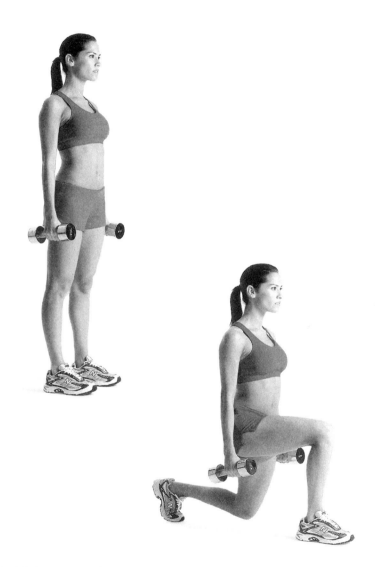

HOME VARIATION: *Use dumbbells, holding one in each hand with your arms at your sides. If you don't have enough space, do the move in one place, alternating your lead foot with each lunge.*

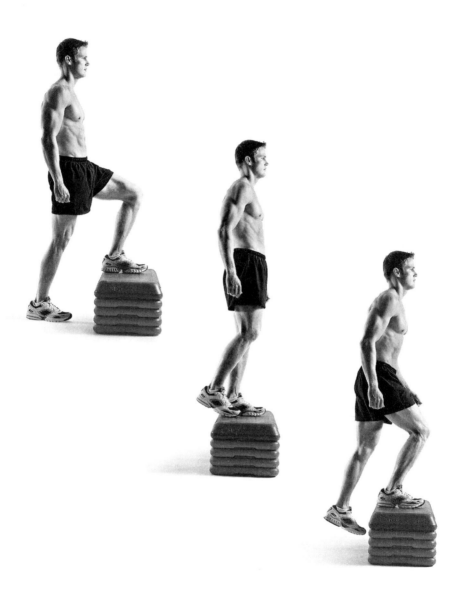

STEP-UP

Use a step or bench that's 18 inches off the ground. Place your left foot on the step so that your knee is bent at 90 degrees. Your knee should not advance past the toes of your left foot. Push down on your left foot, and bring your right foot onto the step, keeping your back straight. Now step down with the left foot, followed by the right. Alternate the leading foot, or do all of the repetitions leading with one foot and then alternating. Once you're comfortable, add dumbbells.

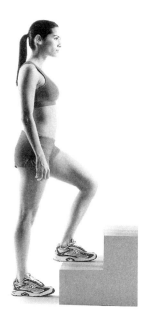

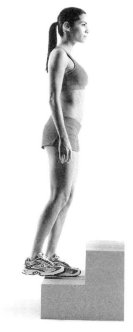

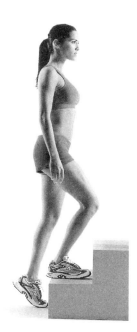

HOME VARIATION:
*Same, only use a staircase instead
of a step if you don't have one.*

The New Abs Diet Interval Workouts

THEY SAY THAT slow and steady wins the race. But the cardiovascular key to fat burning is using interval workouts—workouts that alternate high-intensity levels with lower-intensity effort. Researchers in Canada found that exercisers who did 30-minute workouts that included short, hard bouts of effort lost three times as much fat in 15 weeks as their peers who performed 45-minute-long steady-paced, easier workouts. Interval training, the researchers determined, can increase your cells' ability to burn fat by up to 50 percent. What's more, intervals cause your body to burn calories long after you've stopped exercising. You can use intervals for running, cycling, swimming, on elliptical trainers, even walking if you alternate a speed walk and slow walk. To start, here are three new interval workouts.

INTERVAL VARIATION I: The 20-Minute Sprinter

A typical interval: Switch between bouts of speed and 30-second recoveries.

5 minutes warmup (light jog, low intensity) or until your break a light sweat

10 seconds sprint pace (an 8 to 9 on an intensity scale of 1 to 10)

30 seconds recovery pace (about a 6 on that workout intensity scale)

Repeat this sprint-recovery pattern for 10 minutes

5 minutes cooldown (starting at level 6 in intensity and gradually slowing down until you are walking during the last minute)

Each week, increase the length of the sprint by 5 seconds until you are doing 30-second sprints and 30-second recoveries

INTERVAL VARIATION II: The Pyramid

This pyramid structure allows you to step up to a long bout of peak effort in the middle of the workout and gradually come back down.

3–5 minutes warmup

30 seconds high intensity (7 to 8 on an intensity scale of 1 to 10)

1 minute low intensity (about a 4 in intensity)

||||||||||||||||||||||||||||||||||||||||||||||||||||||||||||||||||||||||||||||||||||||||||||||||||||||

How to Improve Your Cardio Machine Workouts

Cardio machines help you work very hard in a very short period of time, making a morning or lunchtime workout an exercise in efficiency. But most people don't use the machines correctly. Fix your mistakes and you'll get more calorie burn for the effort.

EQUIPMENT	YOUR FORM	YOUR WORKOUT
Treadmill	**The mistake:** Too much bouncing up and down. Your head should remain relatively level while running otherwise you'll tire out your joints—and yourself—too soon. **The fix:** Improve flexibility to smooth out your stride. Try leg swings—with the treadmill off, hold the handlebar, stand on one leg, and swing the other back and forth, keeping your upper body still. Repeat with other leg.	**The mistake:** Too many long, steady, flat runs. **The fix:** Run shorter and harder, mixing speeds and inclines to create intervals. Start with a 2 percent incline, and over several sessions work up to 10 percent. (Just walk at steep inclines.)
Stationary Bike	**The mistake:** The seat is too low or too high. A low seat fatigues the legs and stresses knees. Set it too high and your hips rock from side to side, which is inefficient. **The fix:** Adjust the seat, people! Sit on the seat and place your heel in the middle of the pedal, where the ball of your foot would normally go. You want your leg fully extended, at the lowest point of the pedal rotation. By moving your foot to the correct position on the pedal, you'll have the right amount of bend.	**The mistake:** Cruising instead of charging. **The fix:** Vary the intensity, with 2 to 3 minutes of high-cadence pedaling and a 3-minute recovery, then repeat for 15 minutes. Stand occasionally, which will add another dimension to your workout. Standing requires more muscle not only to push the pedals, but also to support and balance your body.

(chart continues)

EQUIPMENT	YOUR FORM	YOUR WORKOUT
Elliptical Trainer	**The mistake:** Too little resistance. Many people allow momentum to do the work for them instead of propelling the step with their leg muscles. **The fix:** Set the resistance correctly to be able to feel that you are pushing the ramp down when you make a revolution rather than flipping around freely.	**The mistake:** Getting bored. **The fix:** Do intervals. It will force you to reach a higher intensity of training for a sustained period of time. Try 90-second blasts every few minutes, with recoveries twice as long. Reduce recovery time as your fitness level increases.
Stair-climber	**The mistake:** Holding yourself up with your arms. A lot of people put their hands on the railing and lock their elbows with arms straight down. That's like using crutches. **The fix:** Rest your hands lightly on the bars only for balance. Keep your body upright, with just a slight lean forward.	**The mistake:** Too little resistance. **The fix:** Go slower, with challenging resistance. You'll give yourself a tougher workout, increase your heart rate and maintain your time in the training zone longer. **Result:** You'll burn more fat.
Rowing Machine	**The mistake:** Your hands bump your knees, which throws off your cadence. **The fix:** Take a tip from rowing crews to create a fluid motion: Think of the stroke as a dance, counting 1-2-3 and 3-2-1. On 1, push with your legs; on 2, "swing up" your body by leaning back; on 3, draw your arms to the bottom of your rib cage, spinning the flywheel. Then reverse it: 3, extend your arms; 2, swing your body forward from the hips; 1, bring your legs up after the handle passes your knees.	**The mistake:** A long, steady slog, which leads to inefficient exercise. You're spending too much time rowing at a moderate intensity. **The fix:** With medium resistance, do four to six 10-minute sets of high-intensity rowing with 2 to 3 minutes of rest in between. This will allow your heart rate to come down a bit so you can regroup for intense effort. **Result:** You'll expend more calories and get out of the gym quicker.

45 seconds high intensity

1 minute low intensity

90 seconds high intensity

1 minute low intensity

60 seconds high intensity

1 minute low intensity

45 seconds high intensity

1 minute low intensity

30 seconds high intensity

3–5 minutes cooldown

INTERVAL VARIATION III: 15-Minute Rope Burn

I love the jump rope because it's a way to get in a "run" when it's pouring outside and the treadmill is occupied inside. As you know, jumping rope isn't easy. It takes coordination because you're using all your muscles and joints. That's also what makes it such a terrific calorie burner. And a jump rope is an ideal tool for a fast, albeit tough, interval workout. Here's just one rope-jumping interval. Make up more of your own.

5 minutes warmup (easy skipping)

30 seconds high intensity (80 percent of your maximum speed)

1 minute recovery (easy skipping)

30 seconds moderate intensity high-knee skips (lift your knees as high as you can while maintaining an even skip cadence)

1 minute recovery

Continue this pattern for two more circuits

4 minutes alternate between skipping as fast as you can for 60 seconds and easy skipping for 60 seconds

60 seconds cool down (stop rope skipping and walk for 1 minute or until your heart rate returns to normal)

Chapter 13

TARGETING YOUR ABS

A 50-"Six-Pack" of Exercises

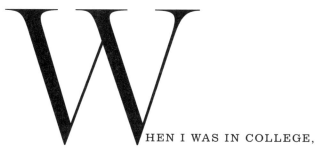HEN I WAS IN COLLEGE, I had a friend who argued that he knew the key to a six-pack: "All you have to do is 1,000 crunches a day for a month." He said it in a way that made you believe him—that if only you were disciplined enough to put in the time every day to concentrate on your abdominal muscles, then you'd eventually chisel away a gut of stone. His theory was that it all boiled down to volume and discipline. He went on to say that the iconic ab exercise would do more than just build abs—that it was also the fix-all to weight problems, that you could simply crunch away years of bingeing on pizza, wings, and all-night keg parties.

In a lot of ways (a heck of a lot of ways, actually), my friend was wrong. For one, crunching won't burn fat. And you won't develop abs by doing the same exercise over and over—let alone the same exercise every day. And 1,000 repetitions? C'mon. There's only one thing most of us would do 1,000 times a day if it were physically possible, and it wouldn't be a crunch. But he was right in one sense: If you want abs that will make you stronger, healthier, and better looking, you do have to work them. And that does take discipline—but not as much as you'd think.

Though your midsection works as one unified core, it does help to think of your abdominal center in regions. To build speed-bump abs, you need to work the entire region. The three visible regions consist of the upper abs, the lower abs, and the obliques (the muscles along the side of your torso). But there are also a number of supporting muscles that, when developed, will add strength to your abdominals: your lower back and the transverse abdominis—muscles that run underneath your abdomen horizontally to give support to your entire midsection.

You already have all of these muscles within you; all you need to do is break them out. That's why your priorities have to revolve around the first two

||||||||||||||||||||||||||||||||||||||||||||||||||||||||||||||||||||||||||||||||||||||||||||||||||||||||||||

Reacquaint Yourself with Your Abs

Your abdominal muscles are a lot like a skilled group of employees. The harder they work, the better they make you look, and vice versa.

This is because you use your abs in virtually every movement that matters. Lifting. Running. Jumping. Reproducing. (It takes a lot of midsection stability to stand over that copy machine. Especially when it's printing on both sides of the page.) So the stronger they are, the harder and longer you'll be able to play. Here's a quick course in the anatomy of your abs.

Rectus abdominis. This is the six-pack muscle that helps your upper body bend (like in a crunch) and also helps keep good posture. It's what people think of when they think of abs.

External obliques. These muscles start on the ribs and extend diagonally down the sides of your waist. If a movement happens at your waist, the external obliques are involved. The torso rotation that's key to golf, tennis, and hockey is mostly a function of the external obliques. Even the basic crunching motion, attributed to the rectus abdominis (the six-pack muscle), wouldn't be possible without a strong contraction of the external obliques to stabilize the torso.

Internal obliques. These lie between the rib cage and the external obliques, and also extend diagonally down the sides of your waist. Similar to the externals, the internal obliques are involved in torso rotation. You use these muscles when you breathe deeply.

Transverse abdominis. It's a thin muscle that runs horizontally, surrounding your abdomen. It's also known as "the girdle" because it functions as a compressor for the abdomen, keeping everything in place.

components: the Abs Diet nutrition principles and the Abs Diet fat-burning workout. Once you strip away the fat from your belly, your abs can grow and show. Unlike what my friend said, you won't find your six-pack by working your abdominal muscles every day. Instead, follow these guidelines for adding the final component:

Work your abs 2 or 3 days a week. Abs are like any other muscle in your body. They'll grow when they're at rest, not when you're working them. So working them every day doesn't give them a chance to grow and get strong. You will develop abs by working them two or three times a week. I'd recommend adding the ab circuit to the beginning of your workout. Saving them until the end of the workout means there's more possibility that you'll skimp and take shortcuts.

Hit the whole region, not just the famed rectus abdominus. (See "Reacquaint Yourself with Your Abs," at left.) You have five regions of your abdominals that you're going to work. For each workout, pick one exercise per region to ensure that you're hitting every area.

Pick different exercises every workout. We're giving you a huge selection exercises for your abdominals, but you need to pick only five exercises each workout. The key is variety: Changing your routine doesn't allow your abs to get comfortable, so they'll continue to grow after each workout.

Do a circuit. In the first week of workouts, just do one set of each exercise (10 to 15 repetitions, depending on the exercise). In the second and third week, do two sets if you'd like, but perform them in a circuit so that you're doing each exercise once before repeating an exercise. After that, you can do three circuits. Even then, your ab workouts shouldn't take more than 5 minutes.

Go slow. Each rep of an ab exercise should last slightly longer than you lasted on prom night—4 to 6 seconds. Any faster, and you run the risk of letting momentum do the work. The slower you go, the higher the intensity. The higher the intensity, the stronger the stomach.

Remember that this portion of the workout is what will make your abs pop out of your skin the way Janet Jackson pops out of her wardrobe. Think of the ab exercise portion of the plan as the toy at the bottom of the cereal box, the paycheck at the end of the week, the finish line at the end of the marathon. It's the motivation. It's the reward. It's the goal that no scale could ever show.

How to Do the Workout

PICK ONE EXERCISE from each group of the listings below, and do the exercise
for the specified number of repetitions. Do one set of each exercise, and then
repeat the circuit.

Note: Many of these exercises target different regions of the abdominals
during the same movement, but they're grouped based on what areas they primarily target. They've also been grouped by levels of difficulty so that you can
change your workouts as you get stronger. For each exercise, pause at the end
of the movement, and return to the starting position. That counts as one repetition, unless otherwise noted.

The Abs Circuit

Upper Abs

Lower Abs

Obliques

Transverse Abdominis

Lower Back

Upper Abs

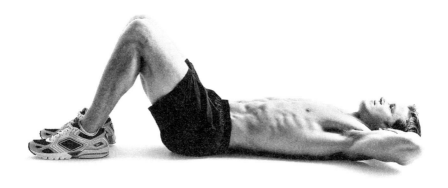

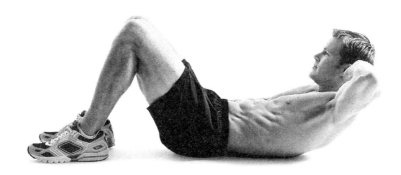

TRADITIONAL CRUNCH

Lie on your back with your knees bent and your hands behind your ears.
Slowly crunch up, bringing your shoulder blades off the ground.

12 to 15 repetitions [*Beginner*]

Upper Abs

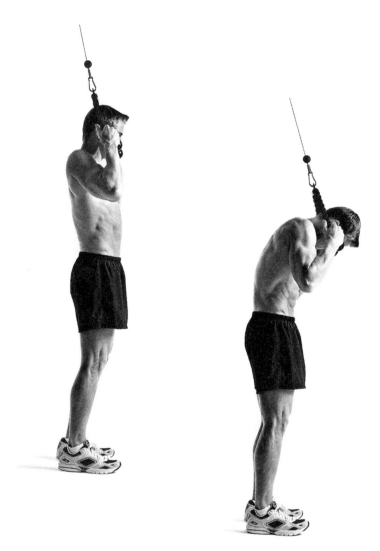

STANDING CRUNCH

Attach a rope handle to a high cable pulley. Stand with your back to the weight stack, and hold the ends of the rope behind your head. Crunch down.

12 to 15 repetitions [*Beginner*]

Upper Abs

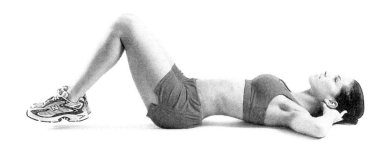

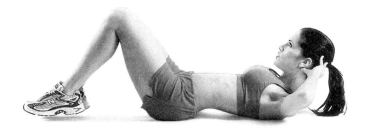

MODIFIED RAISED-FEET CRUNCHES

Lie on your back with your knees bent and your hands behind your ears. Raise your feet just a few inches off the floor, and hold them there. Crunch up, then lower your torso back to the floor, keeping your feet raised throughout the movement.

12 to 15 repetitions [*Beginner to intermediate*]

Upper Abs

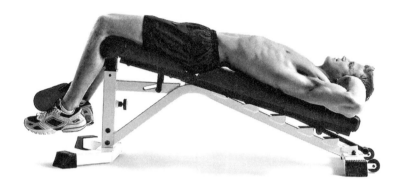

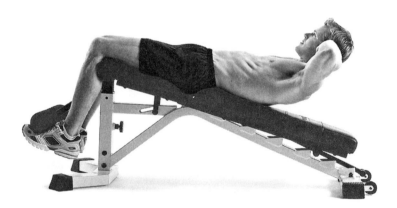

DECLINE CRUNCH

Lie on your back on a decline board, with your ankles locked under the padded support bars and your fingertips cupped behind your ears. Lift your shoulder blades off the bench, keeping your lower body flat. Don't jerk your body to build momentum. Hold the contraction for a second.

12 to 15 repetitions [*Beginner to intermediate*]

Upper Abs

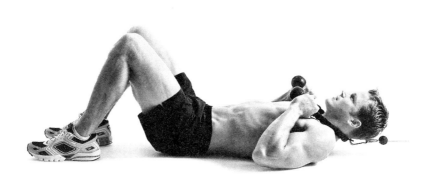

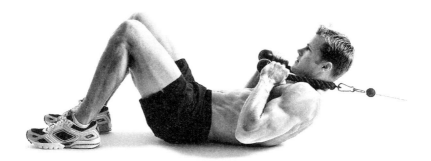

LYING CABLE CRUNCH

Attach a rope handle to the low pulley. Lie on the floor with your head near the low pulley, your knees bent, and your feet flat on the floor. Hold the handle over your chest so that the point of the rope attachment is at the base of your neck. Crunch your rib cage toward your pelvis, lifting your shoulder blades a few inches off the floor.

12 to 15 repetitions [*Intermediate to advanced*]

Upper Abs

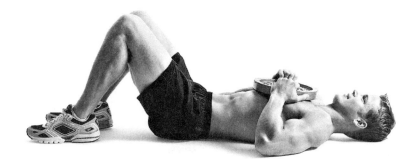

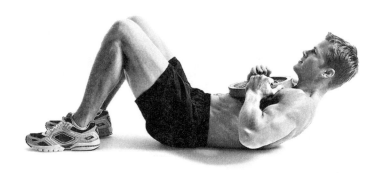

WEIGHTED CRUNCH

Lie on your back with your knees bent, holding a weight plate or dumbbell across your chest. Slowly crunch up, bringing your shoulder blades off the ground. Use progressively heavier weight.

12 to 15 repetitions [*Intermediate to advanced*]

Upper Abs

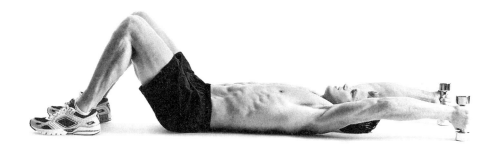

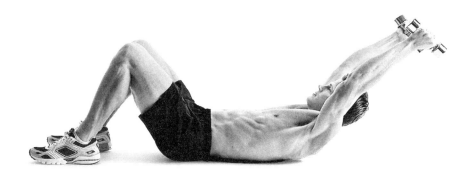

LONG-ARM WEIGHTED CRUNCH

Lie on your back with your knees bent. Hold a light dumbbell in each hand, and stretch your arms straight back behind you. Crunch your rib cage toward your pelvis. Don't generate momentum with your arms.

12 to 15 repetitions [*Intermediate to advanced*]

Upper Abs

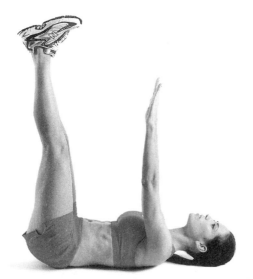

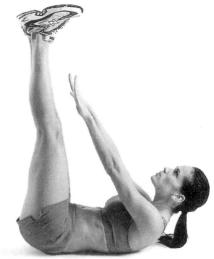

TOE TOUCH

Lie on your back with your legs raised directly over your hips; your knees should be slightly bent. Raise your arms straight up, pointing toward your toes, and relax your head and neck. Use your upper abs to raise your rib cage toward your pelvis, lift your shoulder blades off the floor, and reach toward your toes. Hold for a second. Lower your shoulders to the floor and repeat.

12 to 15 repetitions [*Intermediate to advanced*]

Upper Abs

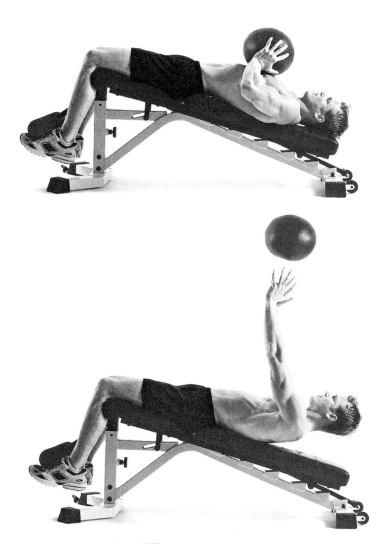

MEDICINE BALL BLAST

Set an adjustable ab bench at a 45-degree angle. Lie down on it with your head toward the floor, and hook your feet under the padded support bars. Hold a medicine ball at your chest as you lower yourself. As you come up, chest-pass the ball straight up over your head. Catch it at the top of the movement, then lower yourself and repeat.

12 to 15 repetitions [*Advanced*]

Upper Abs

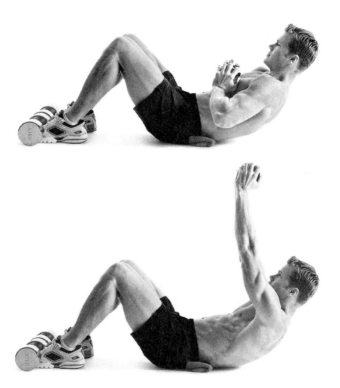

SICILIAN CRUNCH

Slide your feet under the handles of heavy dumbbells. Place a rolled-up towel under your lower back, and hold a dumbbell across your chest. Raise your upper body as high as possible by crunching your rib cage toward your pelvis. At the top of the move, straighten your arms and raise the dumbbell above your head. Keep the dumbbell above your head, and take 4 seconds to lower your body to the starting position.

10 repetitions [*Advanced*]

Lower Abs

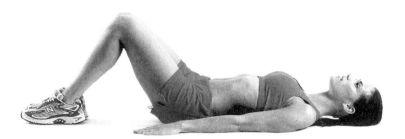

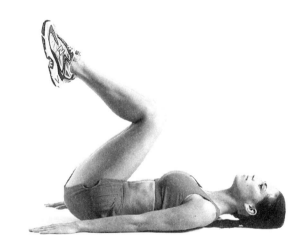

BENT-LEG KNEE RAISE

Lie on your back with your head and neck relaxed and your hands on the floor near your butt. Your feet should be flat on the floor. Use your lower abdominal muscles to raise your knees toward your rib cage, then slowly lower your feet back to the starting position. As your feet lightly touch the floor, repeat.

12 repetitions [*Beginner*]

Lower Abs

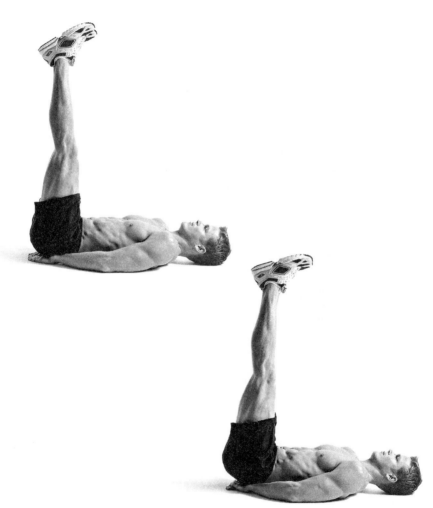

PULSE-UP

Lie with your hands underneath your tailbone and your legs raised and pointed straight up toward the ceiling, perpendicular to your torso. Pull your navel inward, and flex your glutes as you lift your hips just a few inches off the floor. Then lower your hips.

12 repetitions [*Beginner*]

Lower Abs

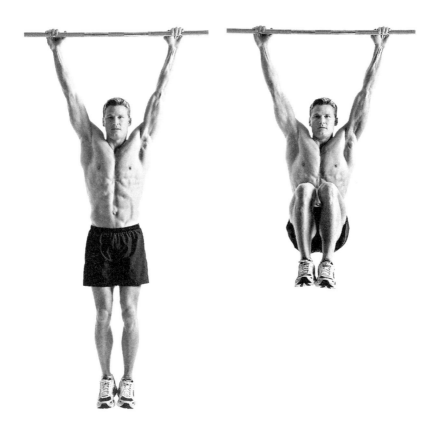

HANGING KNEE RAISE

Hang fully extended from a chinup bar, with your palms facing out and your hands a little farther than shoulder-width apart. (Your feet may lightly touch the floor.) Raise your knees toward your chest, curling your pelvis upward at the end. When you can do that for 12 repetitions, make it tougher by keeping your legs straight as you raise your knees or by holding a medicine ball between your knees.

12 repetitions [*Beginner to intermediate*]

Lower Abs

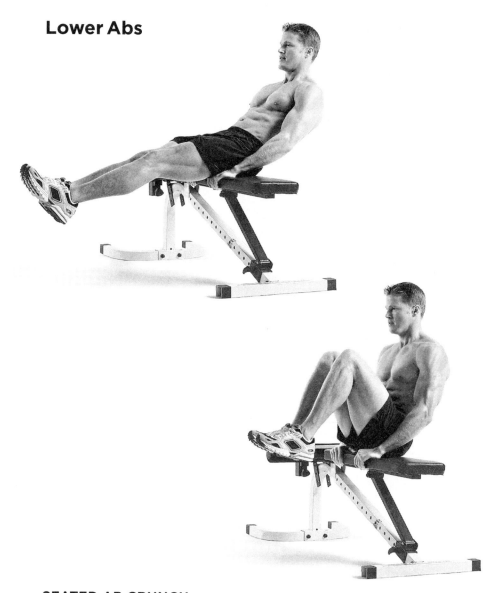

SEATED AB CRUNCH

Sit on the edge of a stable chair or bench. Place your hands in front of your butt, and grip the sides of the seat. Lean back slightly and extend your legs down and away, keeping your heels 4 to 6 inches off the floor. To begin the exercise, bend your knees and slowly raise your legs toward your chest. At the same time, lean forward with your upper body, allowing your chest to approach your thighs.

12 repetitions [*Beginner to intermediate*]

Lower Abs

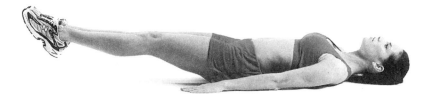

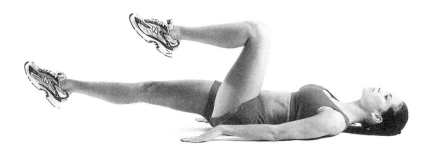

RAISED KNEE-IN

Lie on your back. Your arms should be close to your sides, with your palms down and just under your lower back and butt. Press the small of your back against the floor, and extend your legs outward, with your heels about 3 inches above the floor. Keeping your lower back against the floor, lift your left knee toward your chest. Your right leg should remain hovering above the floor. Hold, then straighten your left leg to the starting position and repeat with your right leg. Keep your abs tight throughout the exercise.

8 to 12 repetitions each side [*Intermediate*]

Lower Abs

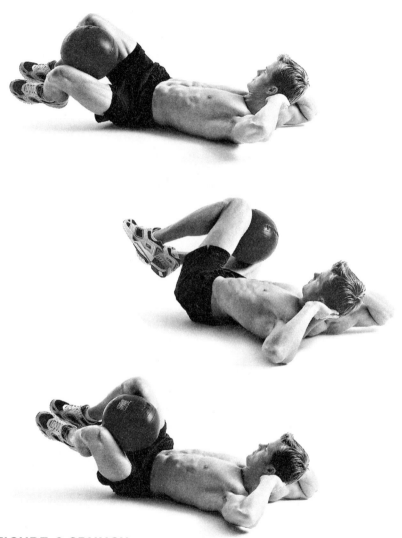

FIGURE-8 CRUNCH

Lie on your back with your knees bent at a 90-degree angle and your feet flat on the floor. Squeeze a light medicine ball tightly between your knees. Cup your hands lightly over your ears, then slowly raise your head, shoulders, and feet off the floor. Move your knees in a wide figure-8 motion. Do three repetitions in one direction, then reverse the motion for three repetitions.

6 repetitions [*Intermediate*]

Lower Abs

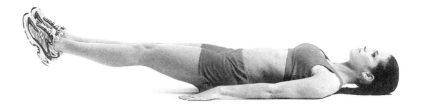

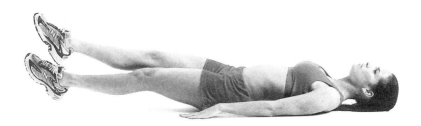

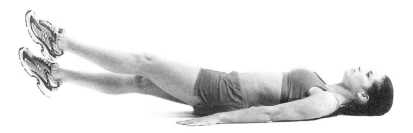

FLUTTER KICK

Lie on your back, raise both feet about a foot off the ground, and scissor-kick one leg over the other.

20 repetitions [*Intermediate*]

Lower Abs

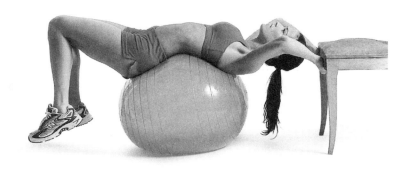

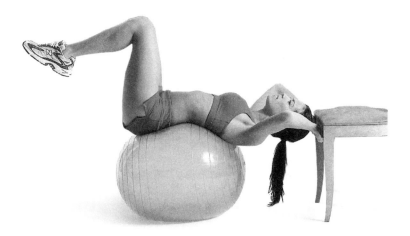

SWISS BALL KNEE RAISE

Lie faceup on a Swiss ball, with your hips lower than your shoulders. Reach back and grab something that won't move, such as a bench or desk. Lift and bend your legs so that your feet are off the floor and the lower parts of your legs point ahead. (To make it more difficult, hold your legs straight out.) Do a standard bent-leg knee raise, using your abs and hip flexors to curl your knees toward your chest.

12 repetitions [*Intermediate to advanced*]

Lower Abs

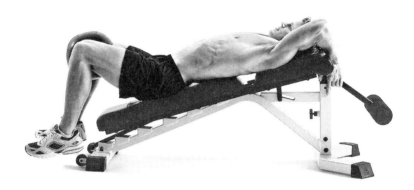

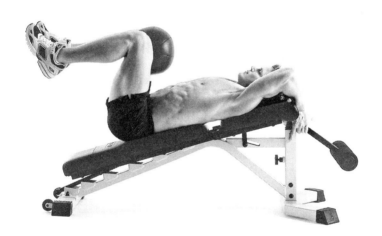

REVERSE CRUNCH HOLDING MEDICINE BALL

Lie on a slant board with your hips lower than your head. Grab the bar behind
your head for support. Bend your hips and knees at 90-degree angles, and hold
a small medicine ball between your knees. Start with your butt flat against the
board. Pull your hips up and in toward your rib cage. Curl them as high as you can
without lifting your shoulders off the board, and keep your hips and knees at
90-degree angles.

12 repetitions [*Intermediate to advanced*]

Lower Abs

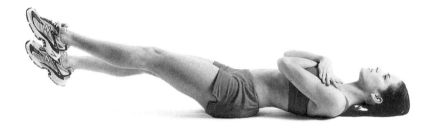

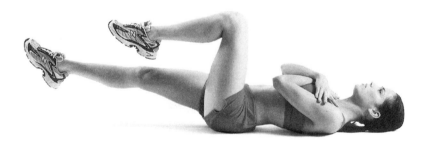

PUSH-AWAY

Lie on your back with your hands on your chest, legs extended, feet raised off the floor. Alternately bring each knee toward your head, then forcefully kick forward. Don't let your feet touch the floor. (If you feel any discomfort in your lower back while performing this exercise, try lifting your head and tucking your chin toward your chest.)

10 repetitions each side [*Intermediate to advanced*]

Obliques

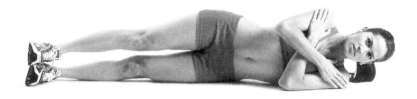

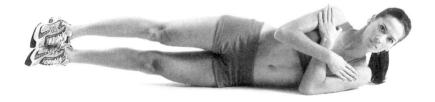

OBLIQUE V-UP

Lie on your side with your body in a straight line. Fold your arms across your chest. Keeping your legs together, lift them off the floor as you raise your top elbow toward your hip. The range of motion is short, but you should feel an intense contraction in your obliques.

10 repetitions each side [*Beginner*]

Obliques

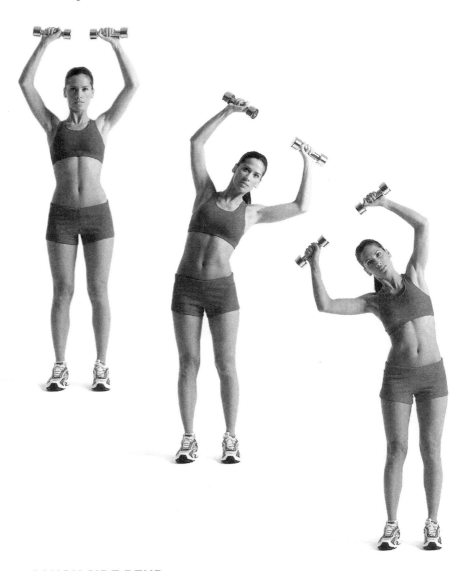

SAXON SIDE BEND

Hold a pair of lightweight dumbbells over your head, in line with your shoulders, with your elbows slightly bent. Keep your back straight, and slowly bend directly to your left side as far as possible without twisting your upper body. Pause, return to an upright position, then bend to your right side as far as possible.

6 to 10 repetitions on each side [*Beginner to intermediate*]

Obliques

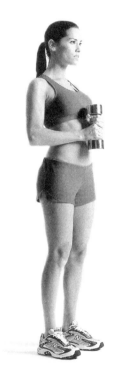
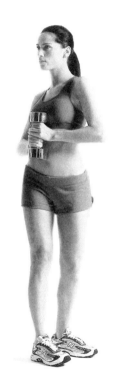

SPEED ROTATION

Stand while holding a dumbbell with both hands in front of your midsection. Twist 90 degrees to the right, then 180 degrees to your left. Keep your abs tight and move fast. Bring to center. Alternate the side you start with.

10 repetitions each side [*Intermediate*]

Obliques

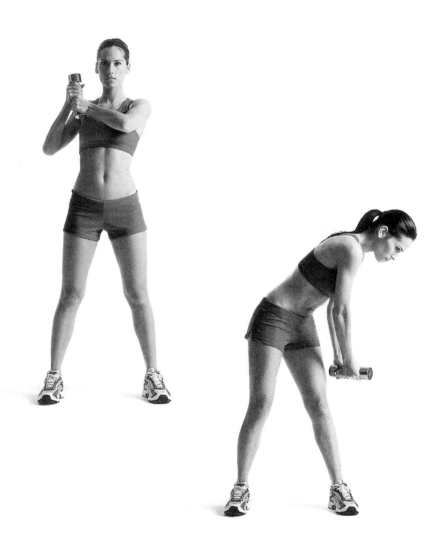

TWO-HANDED WOOD CHOP

Stand while holding a dumbbell, with both hands next to your right ear. Flex your abs and rotate your torso to the left as you extend your arms and lower the dumbbell to the outside of your left knee. Lift it back, finish the set, and repeat on the other side.

10 repetitions each side [*Intermediate*]

Obliques

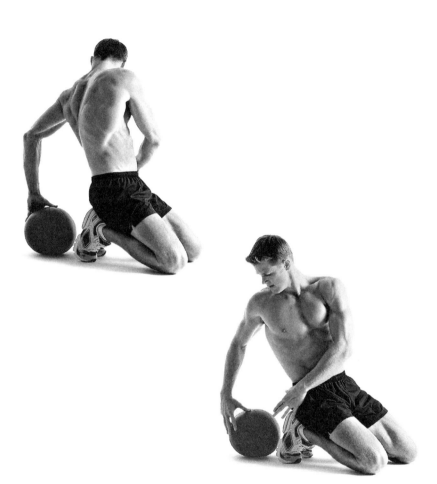

MEDICINE BALL TORSO ROTATION

Hold a medicine ball or basketball in front of you. Sit with your knees bent and your feet on the floor. Quickly twist to your left, and set the ball behind your back. Twist to the right, and pick up the ball. Bring the ball around to your left, and set it down again. Repeat. Do the same number of repetitions in which you first twist to the left side as you do when you twist to the right side.

10 repetitions each side [*Intermediate to advanced*]

Obliques

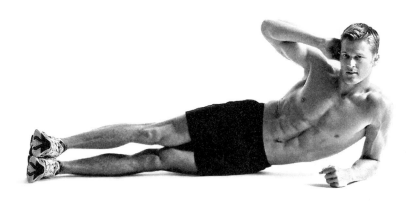

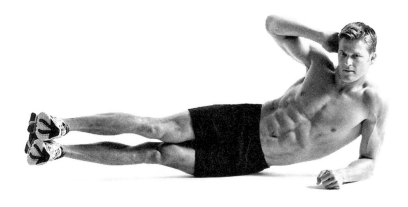

SIDE JACKKNIFE

Lie on your left side with your torso propped up on your left forearm and your legs nearly straight. Hold your right hand behind your right ear, with your elbow pointed toward your feet. While keeping your torso stationary, lift your legs as far as you can. The motion should feel like a crunch—a contraction on the right side of your waist and in your core. Slowly lower your legs and repeat. Finish a set of 10 reps on that side, then repeat on your right side.

10 repetitions each side [*Intermediate to advanced*]

Transverse Abdominis

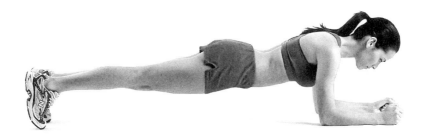

BRIDGE

Start to get in a pushup position, but bend your elbows and rest your weight on your forearms instead of your hands. Your body should form a straight line from your shoulders to your ankles. Pull your abdominals in; imagine you're trying to move your belly button back to your spine. Hold for 20 seconds, breathing steadily. As you build endurance, you can do one 60-second set.

1 to 2 repetitions [*Beginner to intermediate*]

Transverse Abdominis

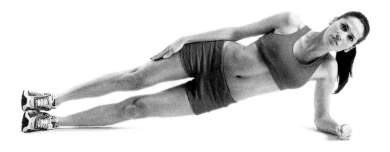

SIDE BRIDGE

Lie on your nondominant side. Support your weight with that forearm and the outside edge of that foot. Your body should form a straight line from head to ankles. Pull your abs in as far as you can, and hold this position for 10 to 30 seconds, breathing steadily. Relax. If you can do 30 seconds, do one repetition. If not, try for any combination of reps that gets you up to 30 seconds. Repeat on your other side.

1 to 2 repetitions on each side [*Beginner to intermediate*]

Transverse Abdominis

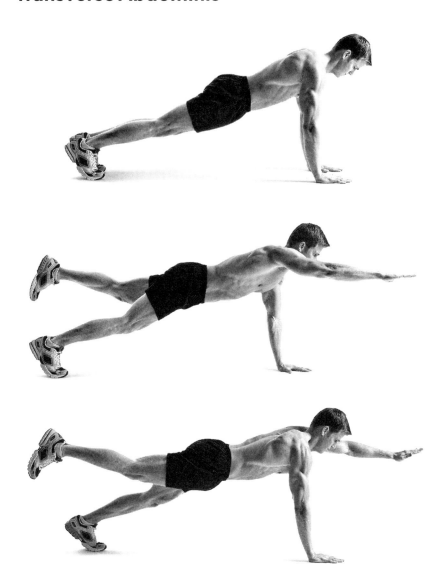

TWO-POINT BRIDGE

Get into the standard pushup position. Lift your right arm and your left leg off the floor at the same time. Hold for 3 to 5 seconds. That's one repetition. Return to the starting position, then repeat, lifting your left arm and right leg this time.

6 to 10 repetitions each side [*Intermediate*]

Transverse Abdominis

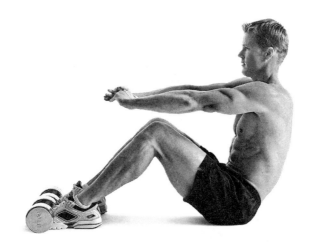

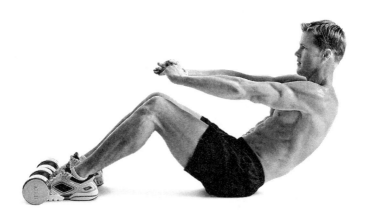

NEGATIVE CRUNCH

Sit on the floor with your knees bent and your feet flat on the floor and shoulder-width apart. Extend your arms with your fingers interlaced, palms facing your knees. Begin with your upper body at slightly less than a 90-degree angle to the floor. Lower your body toward the floor, curling your torso forward, rounding your lower back, and keeping your abs contracted. When your body reaches a 45-degree angle to the floor, return to the starting position. (Note: You may need to tuck your feet under a set of weights to help maintain balance throughout the exercise.)

10 repetitions [*Intermediate*]

Transverse Abdominis

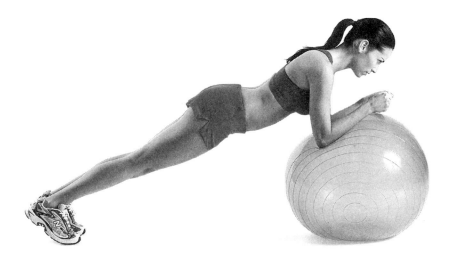

SWISS BALL BRIDGE

Rest your forearms on the ball and your toes on the floor, with your body in a straight line. Pull your stomach in, trying to bring your belly button to your spine. Hold for 20 seconds, breathing steadily. As you build endurance, you can do one 60-second set.

1 to 2 repetitions [*Intermediate to advanced*]

Transverse Abdominis

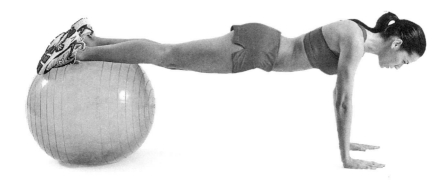

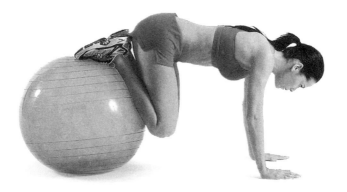

SWISS BALL PULL-IN

Get into the pushup position—your hands set slightly wider than and in line with your shoulders—but instead of placing your feet on the floor, rest your shins on a Swiss ball. With your arms straight and your back flat, your body should form a straight line from your shoulders to your ankles. Roll the Swiss ball toward your chest. Pause, then return the ball to the starting position by extending your legs to the starting position and rolling the ball backward.

5 to 10 repetitions [*Intermediate to advanced*]

Transverse Abdominis

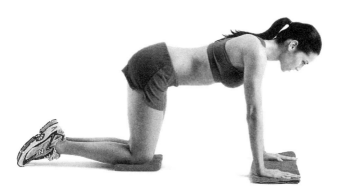

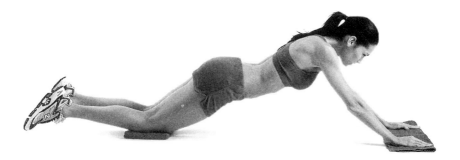

TOWEL ROLL

Kneel on a towel or mat on a tile or wooden floor. Put a towel on the floor in front of you, and place your hands on it. Slide the towel across the floor until your body is fully extended. Your body should look as if you're in a diving position. Slowly slide back up.

5 to 10 repetitions [*Advanced*]

Transverse Abdominis

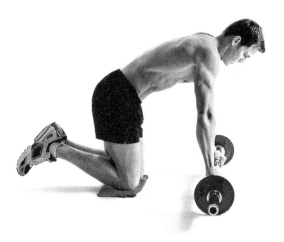

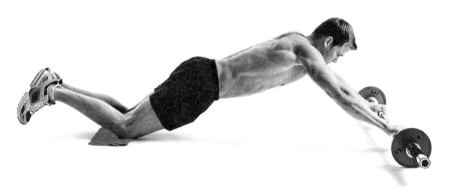

BARBELL ROLLOUT

Load a pair of 5-pound plates into a barbell. Kneel on an exercise mat or towel, with your shoulders directly over the bar. Grab the bar with an overhand, shoulder-width grip. Start with your back in a slightly rounded position, allowing it to extend into a more neutral position as you execute the movement. Roll the bar out in front of you, holding your knees in place as your hips, torso, and arms go forward. Keeping your arms taut, advance as far as you can without arching your back or touching the floor with anything above your knees. Pause for a split second, then pull back to the starting position.

5 to 10 repetitions [*Advanced*]

Lower Back

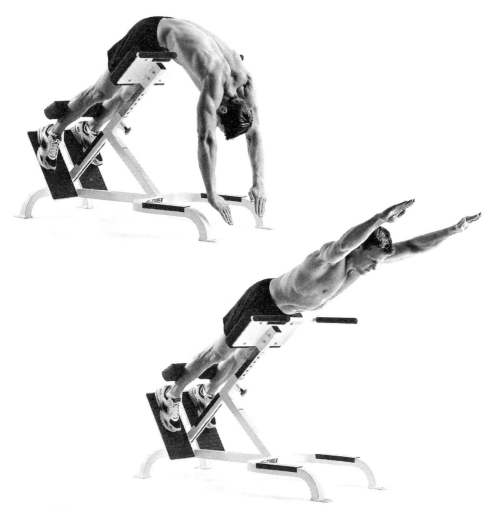

BACK EXTENSION

Position yourself in a back extension station, and hook your feet under the leg anchor. Hold your arms straight out in front of you. Your body should form a straight line from your hands to your hips. Lower your torso, allowing your lower back to round, until it's just short of perpendicular to the floor. Raise your upper body until it's slightly above parallel to the floor. At this point, you should have a slight arch in your back, and your shoulder blades should be pulled together. Pause for a second, then repeat.

12 to 15 repetitions [*Beginner to intermediate*]

Lower Back

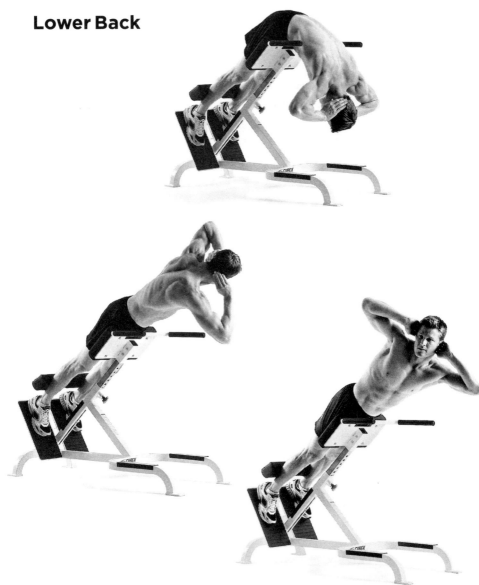

TWISTING BACK EXTENSION

Position yourself in a back extension station, and hook your feet under the leg anchor. Place your fingers lightly behind or over your ears. Lower your upper body, allowing your lower back to round, until it's just short of perpendicular to the floor. Raise and twist your upper body until it's slightly above parallel to the floor and facing left. Pause, then lower your torso and repeat, this time twisting to the right.

12 to 15 repetitions [*Intermediate*]

Lower Back

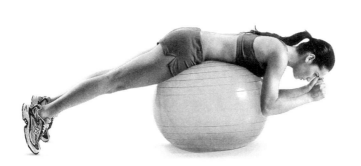

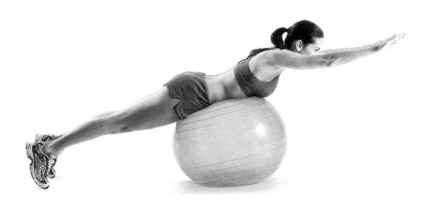

SWISS BALL SUPERMAN

Lie facedown over a Swiss ball so that your hips are pressed against the ball and your torso is rounded over it. Lift your upper arms so that they're parallel to your body, and bend your elbows 90 degrees so that your fingers are pointing forward and your elbows are pointing back. Slowly extend your back until your chest is completely off the ball, extend your arms forward, and hold that position. Draw your arms back into position as you return your torso to the ball.

12 to 15 repetitions [*Intermediate*]

Lower Back

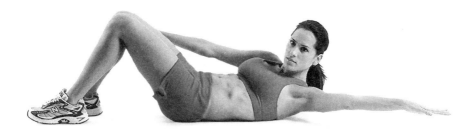

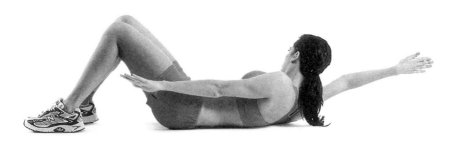

SWIMMER'S BACKSTROKE

Lie faceup on the floor, with your knees bent and feet flat. Flatten your lower back against the floor. Now do a crunch to flex your trunk forward, and lift your shoulder blades as high off the floor as you possibly can. Keeping your chest high, perform a backstroke with one arm at a time, allowing your torso to twist toward the arm that's reaching back. Work up to five repetitions of 45 seconds each, alternating arms. The higher you lift your chest off the floor, the better your exercise will work. Add light dumbbells when the move becomes too easy.

1 to 5 repetitions [*Intermediate to advanced*]

Bonus! The 18 Above-the-Belt Time Savers!

LOOKING TO SHAVE even more time off your workout while shaving fat from your waistline? The remaining 18 moves of our abs plan work several areas of your midsection simultaneously. Use any one of the following substitutions to cover two or three areas with one exercise, and you can reduce your workout plan to just a few exercises instead of five!

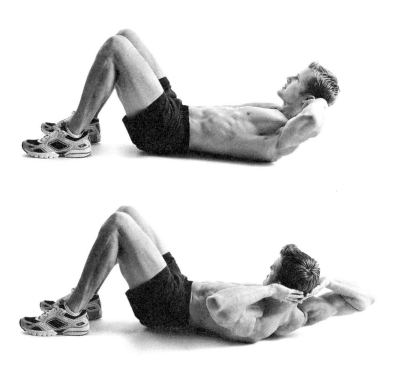

CRUNCH/SIDE BEND COMBO
Targets both the upper abs and obliques
Lie on your back, with your knees bent and your hands behind your ears. Curl up so that your shoulder blades are off the floor. Bend at the waist to the left, aiming your left armpit toward your right hip. Straighten, then bend to your right.

8 repetitions to each side [*Beginner*]

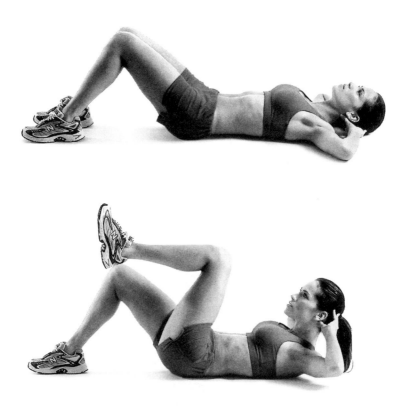

SINGLE-KNEE CRUNCH
Targets both the upper and lower abs
Lie on your back, with your hips bent so your feet are flat on the floor. Touch your fingers to the sides of your head, with your elbows bent. Raise your head, shoulders, and butt off the floor as you simultaneously bring your left knee toward your chest. Lower your torso and leg back down, then repeat the exercise, this time drawing your right knee up as you crunch.

10 repetitions each side [*Beginner to intermediate*]

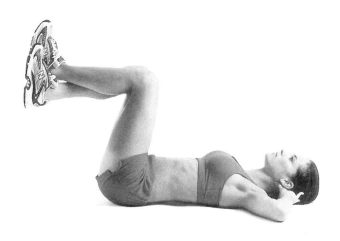

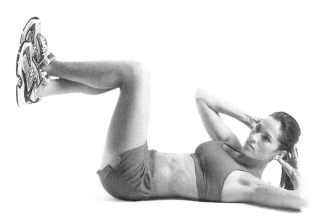

TWISTING CRUNCH
Targets both the upper abs and obliques

Lie on your back on the floor, with your hands cupped behind your ears and your
elbows out. Cross your ankles, with your knees slightly bent, and raise your legs
until your thighs are perpendicular to your body. Bring your right shoulder off the
floor as you cross your right elbow over to your left knee. Return to the starting
position and repeat, beginning with the left shoulder, crossing your left elbow
over to your right knee.

8 repetitions to each side [*Beginner to intermediate*]

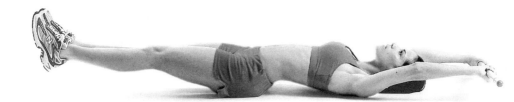

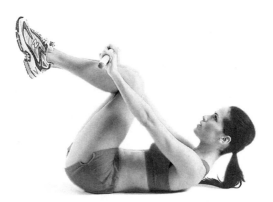

STICK CRUNCH

Targets both the upper and lower abs

Lie on your back, with your feet raised off the ground and your knees slightly bent.
Hold a broomstick behind your head, with your arms extended and off the ground.
Crunch your torso up, and draw your knees and arms inward until the stick extends
past your knees. Pause, then return to the starting position.

12 repetitions [*Intermediate*]

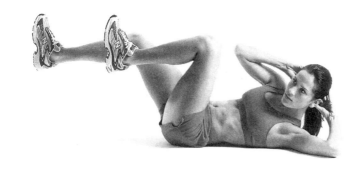

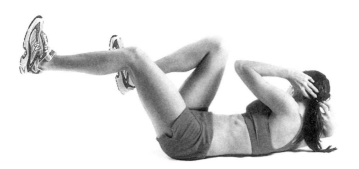

BICYCLE
Targets both the upper and lower abs
Lying on your back with your knees bent 90 degrees and your hands behind your ears, pump your legs back and forth, bicycle-style, as you rotate your torso from side to side by moving an armpit (not an elbow) toward the opposite knee.

20 repetitions [*Intermediate*]

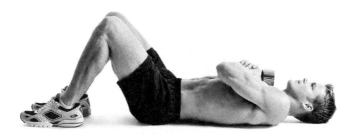

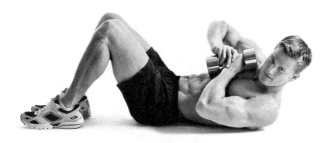

WEIGHTED ONE-SIDED CRUNCH
Targets both the upper abs and obliques

Lie with your knees bent and feet flat on the floor. Hold a dumbbell by your right shoulder with both hands. Curl your torso up and rotate to the left. Lower yourself, finish the set, then repeat, placing the dumbbell next to your left shoulder.

8 repetitions to each side [*Intermediate*]

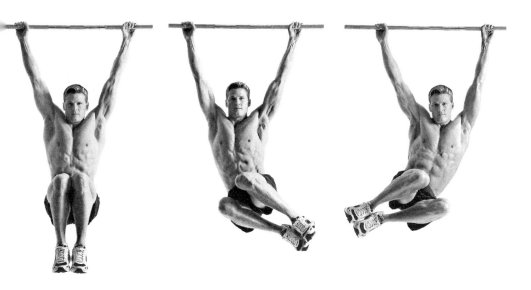

OBLIQUE HANGING LEG RAISE
Targets both the lower abs and obliques

Grasp a chinup bar with an overhand grip and hang from it at arm's length, with your knees bent. Keep your knees bent, and lift your left hip toward your left armpit until your lower legs are nearly parallel to the floor. Pause, then return to the starting position, and lift your right hip toward your right armpit.

10 repetitions each side [*Intermediate*]

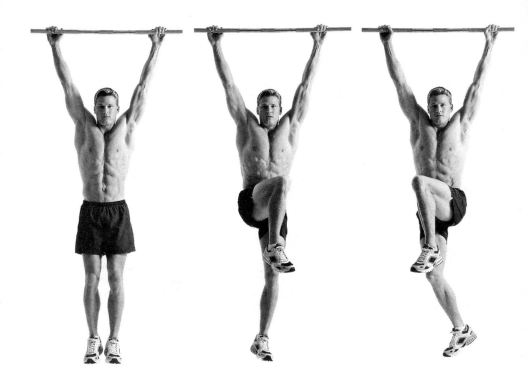

HANGING SINGLE-KNEE RAISE
Targets both the lower abs and obliques

Hang fully extended from a chinup bar, with your palms facing out and your hands a little farther than shoulder-width apart. Your feet should lightly touch the floor. Without swinging to pick up momentum, raise your right knee toward your left shoulder as far as you can, using your abs for power. Slightly thrust your pelvis forward to help, but don't rock. Hold for a second, then lower to the starting position. Repeat with your left leg, raising it toward your right shoulder.

8 to 12 repetitions each side [*Intermediate*]

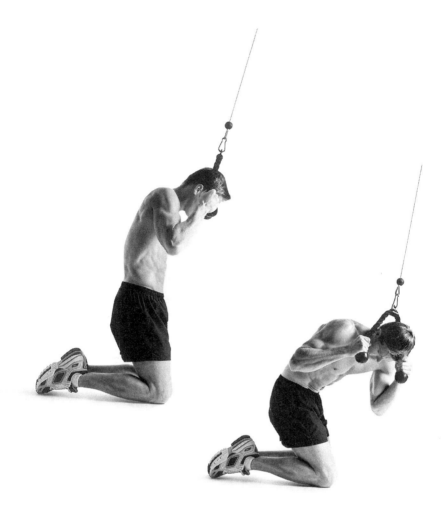

KNEELING THREE-WAY CABLE CRUNCH
Targets both the upper abs and obliques

Attach a rope to the handle of the high pulley. Kneel facing the pulley, and grab the ends of the rope, with your palms facing each other. Hold the rope along the sides of your face, with your elbows slightly bent. Bend forward at the waist, rounding your back and aiming your chest at your pelvis. Stop when you feel a contraction in your abdominal muscles. Return to the starting position, then repeat the movement, this time aiming your chest toward your right knee. Stop when you feel a contraction in your left obliques. Return, then repeat the movement to your left. That's one repetition.

8 repetitions [*Intermediate to advanced*]

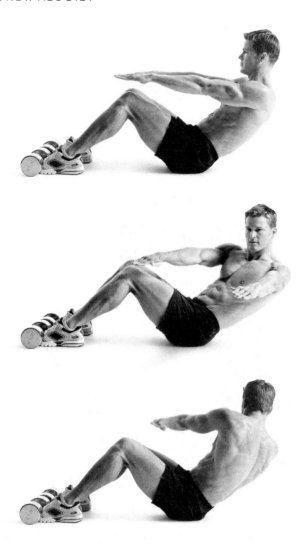

RUSSIAN TWIST
Targets both the upper abs and obliques

Sit on the floor, with your knees bent and your feet flat. Hold your arms straight out in front of your chest, with your palms facing down. Lean back so that your torso is at a 45-degree angle to the floor. Twist to the left as far as you can, pause, then reverse your movement and twist all the way back to the right as far as you can. As you get stronger, hold a light weight in your hands as you do the movement. (Note: You may need to tuck your feet under a set of weights to help maintain balance throughout the exercise.)

10 repetitions each side [*Intermediate to advanced*]

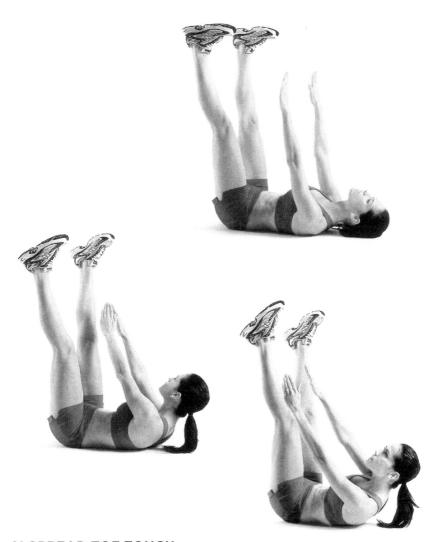

V-SPREAD TOE TOUCH

Targets both the upper abs and obliques

Lie flat on your back, with your legs straight up in a V position without locking your knees. Raise your arms toward the ceiling. Curl your shoulder blades up, and reach toward your right foot with both hands. Hold for a second, concentrating on your abs, then lower to the starting position. Repeat, this time reaching for your left foot. Don't pause at the lower position.

12 to 15 repetitions [*Intermediate to advanced*]

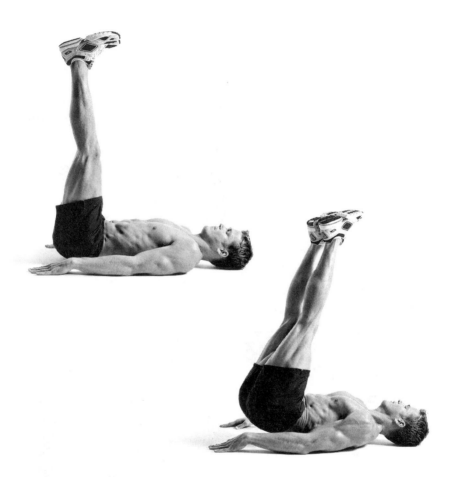

CORKSCREW
Targets both the lower abs and obliques
Lie on your back, with your legs raised directly over your hips; your knees should be slightly bent. Place your hands with the palms down at your sides. Use your lower abs to raise your hips off the floor and toward your rib cage, elevating your hips straight up toward the ceiling. Simultaneously twist your hips to the right in a corkscrew motion. Hold, then return to the starting position. Repeat, twisting to the left.

10 repetitions [*Intermediate to advanced*]

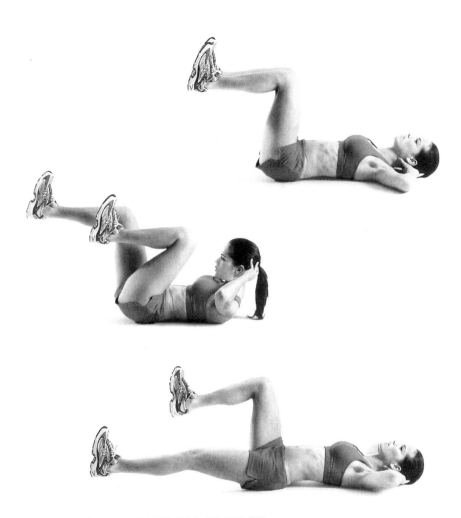

STRAIGHT-LEG CYCLING CRUNCH

Targets both the upper and lower abs

Lie on your back, and bend your hips and knees 90 degrees so that your feet are in the air. Place your hands behind your ears, and perform an abdominal crunch by lifting your head and shoulders off the floor. At the same time, lift your left leg to your chest. Lower your torso to the floor as you straighten your left leg, keeping it a few inches off the floor. Repeat the exercise, this time drawing your right knee up as you crunch. Alternate from left to right throughout the exercise.

10 repetitions each side [Advanced]

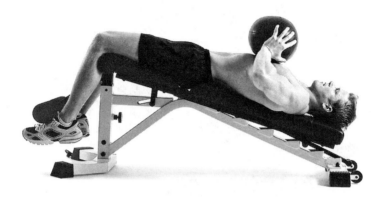

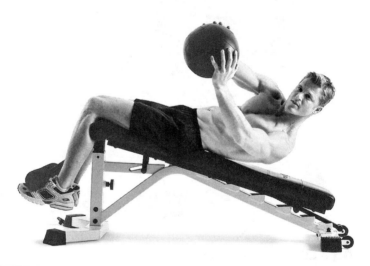

LATERAL MEDICINE BALL BLAST
Targets both the upper abs and obliques

Set an adjustable ab bench at a 45-degree angle. Lie down on it, and hook your feet under the padded support bars. Hold a medicine ball or weight plate against your chest. As you come up, twist to the left and extend your arms as if you were throwing the ball or weight. Pull it back to your chest as you untwist and lower yourself. Repeat, twisting to the right.

5 repetitions each side [*Advanced*]

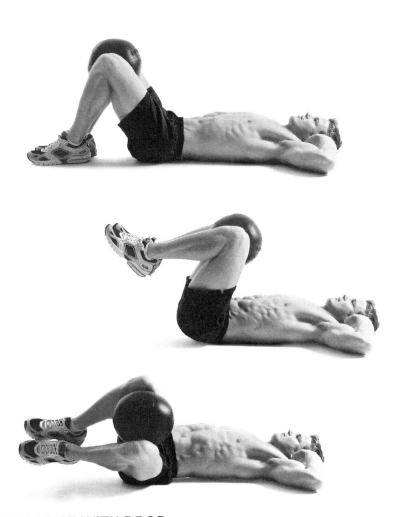

KNEE RAISE WITH DROP
Targets both the lower abs and obliques

Lie on your back, with your hands behind your ears, hips and knees bent, and feet on the floor. Position a medicine ball between your knees. Keep your lower back on the floor throughout the exercise. Contract your abdominals, and pull your knees to your chest. Lower your knees to the left, bring them back to center, then return to the starting position. Drop your knees to the right on the next repetition, and alternate sides for each rep.

12 repetitions [*Advanced*]

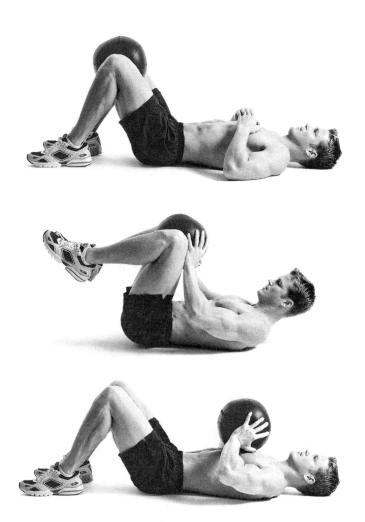

DOUBLE CRUNCH
Targets both the upper and lower abs

Lie on your back, with your hips and knees bent and your feet on the floor. Rest your hands lightly on your chest. Position a medicine ball between your knees. Exhale as you lift your shoulders off the floor and bring your knees to your chest. Grab the ball with your hands, and bring it to your chest as you inhale and return your shoulders and legs to the starting position. Transfer the ball back to your legs on the next repetition, and keep alternating ball positions for the entire set.

12 repetitions [*Advanced*]

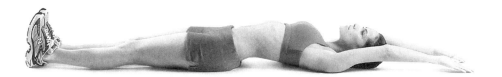

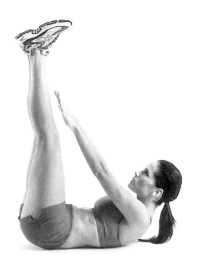

V-UP
Targets both the upper and lower abs
Lie on your back, with your legs and arms extended. Keeping your knees and elbows locked, simultaneously raise your upper body while trying to touch your fingers to your toes.

5 to 10 repetitions [*Advanced*]

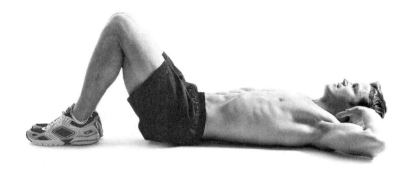

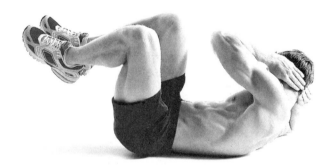

DOUBLE CRUNCH WITH A CROSS
Targets both the upper and lower abs, plus the obliques

Lie on your back with your knees bent, your feet flat on the floor, your head and neck relaxed, and your hands behind your ears. Use your lower abs to lift both knees, and cross them toward your left shoulder as you simultaneously use your upper abs to raise your left shoulder and cross it toward your right knee. Hold for a second. Lower your legs and torso to the starting position, and repeat to the other side.

10 repetitions each side [*Advanced*]

Special Bonus Section

THE ULTIMATE EIGHT-PACK
New Exercises to Upgrade Your Abs

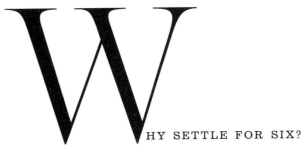

HY SETTLE FOR SIX? You don't have to be an Olympic gymnast to score the ultimate abs trophy— an eight-pack. You can sculpt your own in record time if you eat right, add aerobic exercise to your daily regimen, and use the all-new eight-exercise eight-pack program detailed in this section. As you've learned, your abs are actually one long sheet of muscle called the rectus abdominis. Running horizontally across that sheet of muscle are three tendons that hold the muscle in place over the intestines. Another tendon, called the linea alba, divides the rectus abdominis into two parts, creating four pairs of sections. This actually makes the abdomen an eight-pack—not a six-pack, as most people believe. Of course, how easily your eight-pack emerges has to do with genetics, not just diligent effort. Most people have an eight-pack, but weak tendon divisions don't always define the bottom row. If you're one of the lucky ones with taut tendons, you still need discipline to melt the fat that hides the rectus abdominis. And you need to make the abdominal muscles grow by doing advanced exercises that use weights or positions that keep the resistance high and the repetitions low (8 to 15). The payoff for following this program is a stronger, more stable core that will help you prevent injury and improve your performance in any sporting activity. This workout has four distinct goals:

Goal 1: A flat midsection! Most people, unless they happen to be following the New Abs Diet, challenge their midsections with moves that focus primarily on the upper portion of the rectus abdominis, leaving the lower portion overlooked and underdeveloped. Our eight-pack plan gives equal attention to both segments.

Goal 2: More speed! The lower abdominals play a crucial role in hip flexion, which moves the knees up and forward. Training these abs helps you pump your knees higher for longer periods of time, which adds inches to your stride. You'll cover greater distances at faster speeds.

Goal 3: Better skills! When you swing or throw, you're channeling power up through your midsection and into your upper body. Weak abs can cause a break in this transfer of energy. Strong trunk stabilizers transfer the greatest amount of power every time.

Goal 4: Stamina and balance! Athletes with weak lower abdominals tend to sway at the waist as they run. This creates additional resistance and forces you to expend extra energy to correct your posture. Strong abs help you maintain the best position for efficiency and extra stamina.

The New Abs Diet Eight-Pack Workout Program

To develop an eight-pack, you need to challenge your abs like they're kids in the gifted program at school: Make them work in ways that they never have, so they're challenged, so they don't get bored, and so they'll grow. That means you'll be using a mixture of exercises, equipment, and forms of resistance that you won't find in the Abs Diet 50- "Six-Pack" of abs exercises shown earlier in Chapter 13.

This is a great program to try after you've completed the 6-week New Abs Diet plan—to take your effort to the next level. It's designed as an 8-week program. Each week, you choose an exercise from each of the two sections described. By the end of the program, you'll be doing all of them—in the order given—to bring out a level of muscular separation and growth you can't achieve using traditional, high-repetition ab exercises alone. (For the medicine-ball and pulley exercises, choose a weight that allows you to do the required number of repetitions with good form. You don't want to injure yourself by using more weight than you're ready to handle. That would be a bummer. You'd be better off doing more reps at a slower pace than trying to use a heavy weight.)

YOUR ROUTINE	WEEKS 1-2	WEEKS 3-4	WEEKS 5-6	WEEKS 7-8
Instruction	Create your routine by picking *one* exercise from each section	Create your routine by picking *one* exercise from each section	Create your routine by picking *two* exercises from each section	Create your routine by *doing all* the exercises *in both* sections in the order shown
Sets of each exercise	2	3	2	1
Total number of sets per workout	4 sets	6 sets	8 sets	8 sets
Repetitions per set	8-12	8-12	8-15	8-15
Speed of each repetition	2 seconds up, 2 seconds down	3 seconds up, 3 seconds down	4 seconds up, 4 seconds down	4 seconds up, 4 seconds down
Rest between sets	45-60 seconds	30-45 seconds	15-30 seconds	None
Number of workouts per week	3	3-4	4	5

Section 1

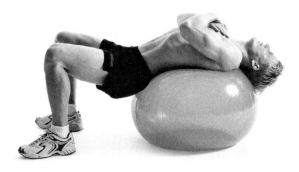

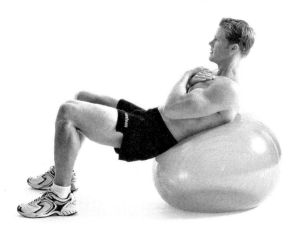

SWISS-BALL CURLUP
Targets both the upper abs and obliques

Recline on a Swiss ball with your head, shoulders, and back in contact with the ball and your feet flat on the floor. Fold your arms across your chest, touching each hand to the opposite shoulder. Pull your belly button in toward your spine to keep your abs tight throughout the move. This helps focus the move more on your abs. Slowly curl your torso up, vertebra by vertebra, stopping just short of an upright seated position. Then lower yourself to the starting position.

WATCH YOUR FORM: *The ball should not move as you curl.*

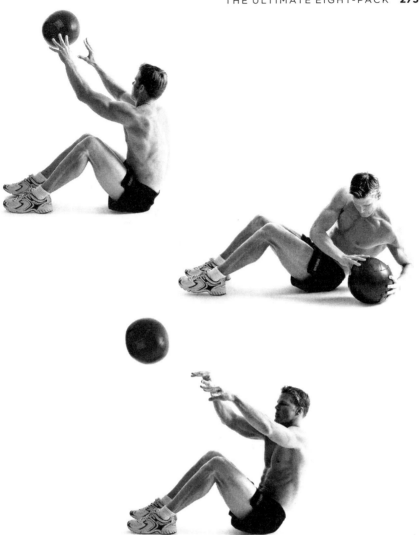

TWISTING MEDICINE-BALL TOSS
Targets both the upper abs and obliques

You'll need a partner. Sit on the floor with your hands in front of your chest, knees bent, feet flat on the floor. Your partner should stand a few feet in front of you and to your right. Have your partner toss a medicine ball toward your right side. Catch it and then twist your body to your left, lowering your torso as you go. Touch the ball to the floor, then toss the ball across your body, back to your partner. After a set, reverse the exercise, with your partner throwing the ball from your left.

WATCH YOUR FORM: *As you throw the ball, try to keep your arms straight.*

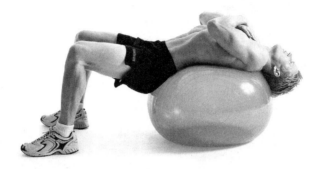

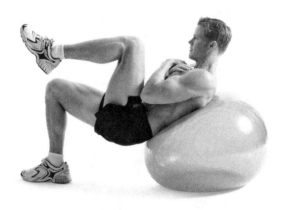

SWISS-BALL CURLUP WITH KNEE TUCK
Targets both the upper and lower abs, plus the obliques

Recline on a Swiss ball, feet flat on the floor, arms crossed on your chest. Your head, shoulders, and back should all be in contact with the ball. Slowly curl your shoulders and upper back up off the ball as you simultaneously draw your left knee toward your chest. Lower your left leg as you lower your torso back down against the ball. Repeat the motion, this time drawing your right knee toward your chest. Continue alternating legs until you've completed all your repetitions.

WATCH YOUR FORM: *Resist the urge to watch your knee move toward your chest.*

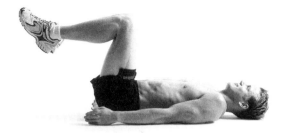

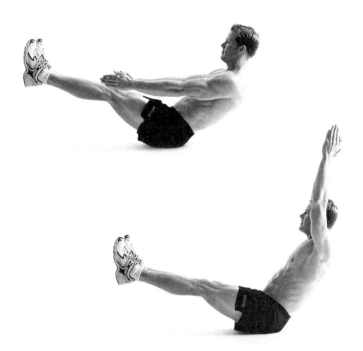

V RAISE

Targets both the upper and lower abs, plus the obliques

Lie on your back with your knees bent at 90 degrees and your feet raised so your thighs are perpendicular to the floor. Slowly extend your legs so they're at a 45-degree angle from the floor as you raise your upper body so your torso is also at 45 degrees. Extend your arms straight out in front of you. Pause, then slowly raise your arms up and back over your head until they're in line with your upper body. Lower your arms so they're parallel to the floor, and return to the starting position.

WATCH YOUR FORM: *If balancing is difficult, raise your arms only as high as you can.*

Section 2

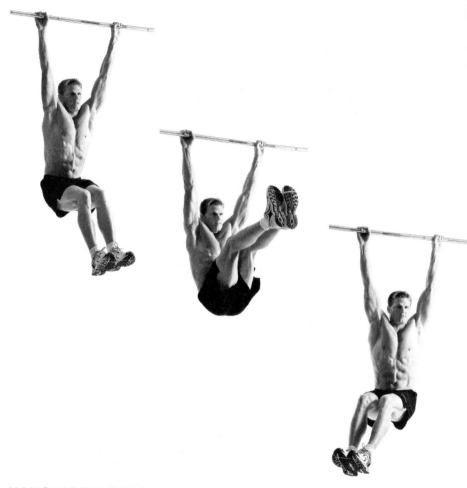

HANGING REVERSE TRUNK TWIST
Targets both the upper and lower abs, plus the obliques
Hang from a pullup bar with your hands shoulder-width apart and your legs slightly bent. Now, raise your legs in front of you until your thighs are parallel to the floor. Pause, then engage your core muscles to tilt your pelvis up and slowly raise your thighs toward your chest as far as you can go (middle photo). Lower your legs slowly until your thighs are once again parallel with the floor. From here, rotate your knees to the right by twisting your hips and keeping your upper body straight. Pause, then rotate the knees to the left as far as you can. Bring your legs back to the center and lower them to the starting position. Repeat.

WATCH YOUR FORM: *Think about tilting your pelvis up, then lifting your legs.*

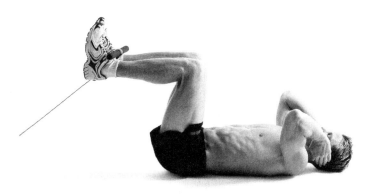

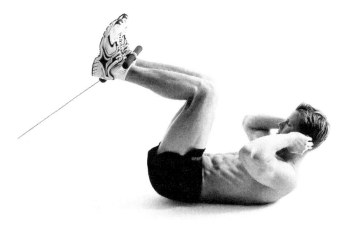

SINGLE-RESISTANCE DOUBLE CRUNCH
Targets both the upper and lower abs

Attach a bar to a low-pulley cable. Sit facing the pulley. Place the cable between your feet so that the bar rests across your insteps. Rest your head and back flat on the floor, bend your knees at a 90-degree angle, and position your thighs perpendicular to the floor. Keeping your legs at a 90-degree angle, slowly curl your head and shoulders off the floor as you tilt your pelvis and curl your legs toward your chest. Pause, then return to the starting position.

WATCH YOUR FORM: *Try to curl your lower body forward to roll your butt off the floor.*

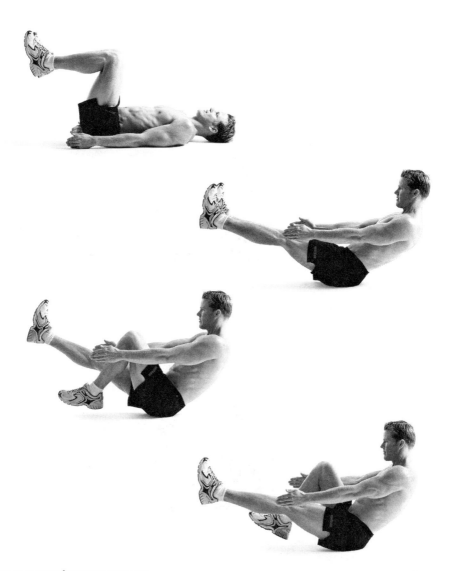

V RAISE/KNEE TUCK

Targets both the upper and lower abs, plus the transverse abdominals

Lie faceup on the floor with your knees bent at 90 degrees and your feet raised so your thighs are perpendicular to the floor. Slowly extend your legs so they're at a 45-degree angle from the floor and simultaneously raise your upper body so your torso is also at 45 degrees. Extend your arms straight out in front of you. Holding this position, slowly draw your left knee in to your chest, then extend it back out. Repeat the motion with your right leg. Continue to alternate legs.

WATCH YOUR FORM: *Go slowly. Imagine that each foot is resisting something heavy.*

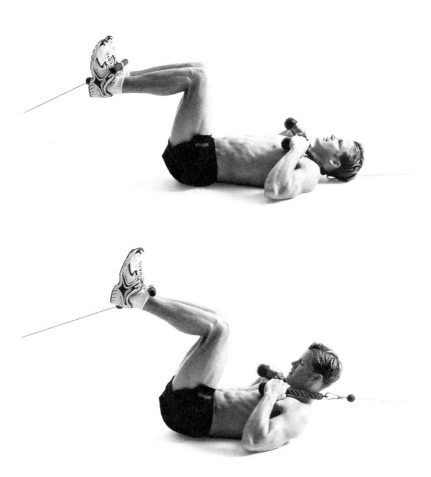

DOUBLE-RESISTANCE DOUBLE CRUNCH
Targets both the upper and lower abs

Attach a rope to one of the low pulley cables and a bar to the other low cable. Lie flat on your back with your head pointing toward the rope and your feet toward the bar. Place the bar on the tops of your shoes so the cable is between your feet. Reach back, grab both ends of the rope, and pull your fists to your chest. Slowly curl your torso up as you simultaneously tilt your pelvis and curl your legs toward your chest. Hold for a second, then slowly lower yourself.

WATCH YOUR FORM: *Try to resist the urge to pull the rope with your arms.*

THE NEW ABS DIET MAINTENANCE PLAN

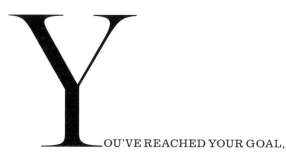

OU'VE REACHED YOUR GOAL, and that's reason to celebrate. But it doesn't give you license to go back to breakfasts of leftover jalapeño poppers. However, you have earned a reprieve. You've built your body to churn fat and build lean muscle. With that base, you're at the point where your body is doing a lot of the work for you. Here's a primer for maintaining the body you've built.

SUBJECT	GUIDELINE
Diet basics	You've adjusted well, and you can continue eating six meals a day by focusing on the Powerfoods—and the super ingredients, like protein, fiber, and whole-grain carbohydrates. Keep drinking smoothies regularly and adding a source of protein to every snack.
Cheating	You can up your cheating meal to a cheating day where you treat yourself to anything you want. Just keep it confined to 1 day rather than spreading it out over several meals on several days. That will increase the chances you'll stay focused and maintain good eating habits.

(continued)

SUBJECT	GUIDELINE
Exercise program	You're in maintenance mode now. Keep going with the program if you like, but you can also scale back to 1 or 2 days a week of strength training and 1 day a week of interval training. Research at the human performance laboratory at Ball State University has shown that lifters can maintain their muscle with just one workout a week.
Abdominal workout	Do a circuit of abdominal exercises before your strength training workouts. Move up to advanced exercises. Now that you can see your abs, you will want to increase the intensity. Still, for maximum growth, you shouldn't work your abs more than 2 or 3 days a week.

NUTRITIONAL VALUES OF COMMON FOODS

T HE NEW TREND TOWARD low-carb diets has a lot of us eating plenty of fat and protein. But many of us are missing out on the valuable micronutrients found in whole grains, fruits, vegetables, and other foods that are verboten on a low-carb diet.

It might seem easier to ensure your daily value of nutrients by popping a multivitamin instead of eating a balanced diet. But there are two problems with nutrition that comes in a plastic container: First, multivitamins have no fiber, so this critical nutrient is missing if all you do is pop a pill for protection. Second, foods are loaded with plenty of nutrients beyond the standard vitamins C and E—and the importance of many of these nutrients, called phytochemicals, is only now being understood. "In a balanced diet, there are thousands of antioxidants. In pill form, you're just getting a few out of the thousands," says Edgar Miller, MD, PhD, of Johns Hopkins University in Baltimore.

To see how nutritionally complete your diet is, refer to the accompanying chart for each food's vitamin and mineral values, and tally up your total intake. If you come up short of the recommended dietary allowances (RDAs)? Don't worry. Just eat more foods high in whatever vitamins or minerals you're lacking.

	VITAMIN A (MCG)	VITAMIN B₁ (THIAMIN) (MG)	VITAMIN B₆ (MG)	FOLATE (MCG)	VITAMIN ((MG)
RDAS FOR MEN/WOMEN	900/700	1.2/1.1	1.3/1.3	400/400	90/75
Almonds (1 ounce)	0	0.05	0.03	11	0
Apple (1 medium)	8	0.02	0.06	4	6
Apricot (1)	67	0.01	0.02	3	3.50
Artichoke (1 medium)	0	0.10	0.15	87	15
Asparagus (1 medium spear)	12	0.02	0.01	8	1
Avocado (1)	122	0.20	0.60	124	16
Bacon (3 slices)	0	0.08	0.07	0.40	0
Bagel (4")	0	0.15	0.05	20	0
Banana (1 medium)	7	0.04	0.40	24	10
Beans, baked (1 cup)	13	0.40	0.34	61	8
Beans, black (1 cup cooked)	1	0.40	0.12	256	0
Beans, kidney (1 cup cooked)	0	0.28	0.21	230	2
Beans, lima (½ cup cooked)	32	0.12	0.16	22	9
Beans, navy (1 cup cooked)	0.36	0.40	0.30	255	1.64
Beans, pinto (1 cup cooked)	0	0.17	0.16	294	1.37
Beans, refried (1 cup)	0	0.07	0.36	28	15
Beans, white (1 cup cooked)	0	0.20	0.17	145	0
Beef, ground lean (3 ounces)	0	0.06	0.24	7	0
Beer (12 ounces)	0	0.02	0.18	21	0
Beets (½ cup)	3	0.02	0.05	74	3
Blueberries (1 pint)	17	0.11	0.15	17	28
Bran, wheat (1 cup)	0	0.14	0.35	14	0
Bread, rye (1 slice)	0.26	0.14	0.02	35	0.13
Bread, white (1 slice)	0	0.11	0.02	28	0
Bread, whole grain (1 slice)	0	0.11	0.10	30	0.08

VITAMIN E (MG)	CALCIUM (MG)	MAGNESIUM (MG)	POTASSIUM (MG)	SELENIUM (MCG)	ZINC (MG)	CALORIES
15/15	1,000/1,000	420/320	3500/3500	55/55	11/8	
6	71	86	180	0	1	170
0.25	8	7	148	0	0.06	80
0.30	5	3.50	90	0.03	0.07	20
0.24	56	77	474	0.26	0.60	25
0.18	4	2	32	0.37	0.10	5
3	22	78	1,204	0.80	0.84	250
0.06	2	6	107	12	0.70	110
0.04	16	26	90	28	1	247
0.12	6	32	422	1	0.20	110
1.35	127	81	752	12	4	239
0.14	46	120	610	2	1.90	240
0.05	62	74	717	2	1.80	260
0.12	27	63	485	1.70	0.70	229
0.73	127	107	670	11	1.90	255
1.61	72	70	495	19	1.70	245
0	88	83	675	3	3	240
1.74	161	113	1,004	2.30	2.50	249
0.15	7	19	265	0	4	185
0	18	21	89	2.50	0.04	153
0.03	11	16	221	0.50	0.24	29
1.65	17	17	223	0.30	0.50	165
0.54	26	220	426	28	3	120
0.11	23	13	53	10	0.36	83
0.06	38	6	25	4.30	0.20	67
0.09	24	14	53	8	0.30	65

	VITAMIN A (MCG)	VITAMIN B₁ (THIAMIN) (MG)	VITAMIN B₆ (MG)	FOLATE (MCG)	VITAMIN (MG)
RDAS FOR MEN/WOMEN	900/700	1.2/1.1	1.3/1.3	400/400	90/75
Breakfast sandwich, fast-food (bacon, egg, and cheese)	0	0.53	0.16	73	2
Brussels sprouts (½ cup)	60	0.08	0.14	47	48
Cake, coffee (1 piece)	20	0.10	0.03	27	0.11
Cake, frosted (1 piece)	10	0.01	0.02	7	0.04
Canadian bacon (2 slices)	0	0.40	0.20	2	0
Candy, nonchocolate (1 package)	0	0	0	0	0
Cantaloupe (1 medium wedge)	345	0.04	0.07	21	37
Carrot (1)	734	0.04	0.08	12	4
Cauliflower (1 cup)	2	0.06	0.22	57	46
Celery (1 cup, strips)	55	0.03	0.10	45	4
Cereal, whole grain, with raisins (½ cup)	3	0.16	0.10	22	0.55
Cheddar cheese (1 slice)	75	0.01	0.02	5	0
Chef's salad with no dressing (1½ cups)	146	0.40	0.40	101	16
Cherries, sweet, raw (1 cup)	30	0.07	0.05	5.80	10
Chicken, skinless (½ breast)	4	0.04	0.32	2	0.71
Chickpeas (1 cup cooked)	4	0.19	0.22	282	2
Chili with beans (1 cup)	87	0.12	0.30	59	4
Chips, potato, light (1 ounce)	0	0.05	0.22	8	3.40
Chocolate (1.45 ounces)	20	0.05	0.01	5	0
Cinnamon bun (1)	0	0.12	0	17	0.06
Citrus fruits and frozen concentrate juices (12 ounces)	7	0.17	0.30	31	324
Clams, fried (¾ cup)	101	0.11	0.07	41	11.25
Coffee (1 cup)	0	0	0	5	0
Collards (1 cup cooked)	1,542	0.08	0.24	177	35

VITAMIN E (MG)	CALCIUM (MG)	MAGNESIUM (MG)	POTASSIUM (MG)	SELENIUM (MCG)	ZINC (MG)	CALORIES
15/15	**1,000/1,000**	**420/320**	**3500/3500**	**55/55**	**11/8**	
0.60	160	25	211	36.0	2	441
0.34	28	16	247	1.17	0.26	28
0.11	76	10	63	9	0.25	180
O	18	14	84	1.40	0.30	239
0.16	5	10	181	11	0.80	137
O	O	O	O	O	O	230
0.05	9	12	272	0.40	0.18	24
0.40	20	7	195	0.06	0.15	35
0.08	22	15	303	0.60	0.30	25
0.33	50	14	322	0.50	0.16	17
0.40	33	70	207	10	1	195
0.08	204	8	28	4	0.90	114
O	235	49	401	37	3	267
0.20	21	16	325	0.90	0.09	90
0.08	6.50	16	150	11	0.50	130
0.60	80	79	477	6	2.50	269
1.46	120	115	934	3	5	220
0.62	10	18	285	2	0.17	142
0.83	78	26	153	2	0.83	230
0.48	10	3.60	19	5	0.10	418
0.24	85	68	1,336	1	0.41	186
O	71	16	366	33	1.60	560
0.05	2	5	114	O	0.02	2
1.67	266	38	220	1	0.50	61

	VITAMIN A (MCG)	VITAMIN B₁ (THIAMIN) (MG)	VITAMIN B₆ (MG)	FOLATE (MCG)	VITAMIN (MG)
RDAS FOR MEN/WOMEN	900/700	1.2/1.1	1.3/1.3	400/400	90/75
Cookie, chocolate chip (1)	0.04	0.01	0.01	0.90	0
Corn (1 cup)	0.26	0.06	0.16	115	12
Cottage cheese, low-fat (1 cup)	25	0.05	0.15	27	0
Crackers (12)	0	0.17	0	0	0
Cranberry juice cocktail (1 cup)	1	0.02	0.05	0	90
Cream cheese (1 tablespoon)	53	0	0	2	0
Cucumber with peel (½ cup)	10	0.01	0.02	7	2.76
Doughnut (1)	17	0.10	0.03	24	0.09
Egg, whole (1 large)	84	0.03	0.06	22	0
Eggplant (1 cup)	4	0.08	0.09	14	1
English muffin, whole wheat (1)	0.09	0.25	0.05	36	0
Fig bar cookies (2 bars)	3	0.05	0.02	11	0.10
Fish, white (1 fillet)	60	0.26	0.50	26	0
French fries (10)	0	0.07	0.16	8	6
Fruit, dried (1 ounce)	208	0.01	0.05	1.1	1
Fruit juice, unsweetened (1 cup)	0	0.02	0.06	35	40
Garlic (1 clove)	0	0	0.04	0.09	0.90
Graham cracker (1 large rectangular piece)	0	0.03	0.01	6	0
Granola bar (1)	2	0.06	0.02	6	0.22
Grape juice (1 cup)	1	0.07	0.16	8	0.25
Ham (1 slice)	0	0.20	0.10	1	0
Hamburger, fast-food, with condiments and vegetables (1)	4	0.30	0.12	52	2
Hot dog, fast-food (1)	0	0.44	0.09	85	0.09
Ice cream (1 serving)	6	0.03	0.04	11	0.46
Jam or preserves (1 tablespoon)	0.20	0	0	2	2

VITAMIN E (MG)	CALCIUM (MG)	MAGNESIUM (MG)	POTASSIUM (MG)	SELENIUM (MCG)	ZINC (MG)	CALORIES
15/15	1,000/1,000	420/320	3500/3500	55/55	11/8	
0.26	2.50	3	14	0	0.06	63
0.15	8	44	343	1.54	1.36	120
0.02	138	11	194	20	0.86	180
0	28	12	48	2.40	0.20	155
0	8	5	46	0	0.18	137
0.04	12	1	17	0.40	0.10	51
0	7	6	75	0	0.10	8
0.90	21	9	60	4	0.30	230
0.50	25	5	63	15	0.50	74
0.40	6	11	122	0.10	0.12	35
0.26	101	21	106	17	0.61	134
0.21	20	9	66	1	0.12	111
0.39	51	65	625	25	2	168
0.12	4	11	211	0.20	0.20	100
0.31	11.82	11.13	226	0	0.14	69
0	160	9	154	0	0.20	117
0	5	0.75	12	0.40	0	4
0.05	3	4	19	1	0.10	59
0.32	15	24	82	4	0.50	117
0	23	25	334	0.25	0.13	154
0.10	2	5	94	6	0.50	30
0.42	126	23	251	20	2	512
0.10	108	27	190	29	2	242
0	72	19	164	1.65	0.40	133
0	4	0.80	15	0.40	0	56

	VITAMIN A (MCG)	VITAMIN B₁ (THIAMIN) (MG)	VITAMIN B₆ (MG)	FOLATE (MCG)	VITAMIN C (MG)
RDAS FOR MEN/WOMEN	900/700	1.2/1.1	1.3/1.3	400/400	90/75
Kale (1 cup)	955	0.07	0.11	18	33
Ketchup (1 tablespoon)	7	0	0.02	2	2
Kiwifruit (1 medium)	3	0.02	0.07	19	70
Lasagna, meat (7 ounces)	61	0.19	0.20	16	12
Lentils (1 cup cooked)	4.75	0.33	0.35	358	0.22
Lettuce, iceberg (1 cup)	8	0.02	0.03	31	2
Lettuce, romaine (½ cup)	81	0.02	0.02	38	7
Liver, beef (3 ounces)	8,042	0.16	0.86	215	1.62
Lunchmeat, salami (3 slices)	0	0.10	0.08	0.34	0
Macaroni and cheese (8 ounces)	48	0.25	0	0	0
Meat loaf (1 slice)	20	0.10	0.14	12	0.62
Melon, honeydew (1 cup)	5	0.07	0.16	34	32
Milk, fat-free (1 cup)	5	0.10	0.10	12	2
Milk, soy (1 cup)	0	0.15	0.16	40	0
Muffin, blueberry (1)	13	0.10	0.01	42	0.63
Mushrooms (1 cup sliced)	0	0.09	0.10	12	2
Nachos with cheese (6–8)	170	0.20	0.20	12	1
Nectarine (1)	23	0.05	0.03	7	7
Oatmeal (1 cup)	0.12	0.12	0.10	13	0
Olives (1 tablespoon)	1.70	0	0	0	0
Onion rings (10 medium)	0.98	0.10	0.07	64	0.68
Oyster (1 medium)	4.20	0.01	0.01	1.40	0.52
Pancakes (2)	7.60	0.16	0.07	28	0.15
Pasta with red sauce (4.5 ounces)	0	0.13	0.10	4	6
Peach (1 medium)	16	0.02	0.02	4	6
Peanut butter (2 tablespoons)	0	0.03	0.15	24	0
Peanuts (1 ounce)	0	0.12	0.07	41	0

VITAMIN E (MG)	CALCIUM (MG)	MAGNESIUM (MG)	POTASSIUM (MG)	SELENIUM (MCG)	ZINC (MG)	CALORIES
15/15	**1,000/1,000**	**420/320**	**3500/3500**	**55/55**	**11/8**	
1	180	23	417	1.17	0.23	39
0.20	3	3	57	0.04	0	15
1	26	13	237	0.15	0.10	50
0.94	220	41	372	28	3	318
2.97	37	71	731	5.54	2.51	230
0.02	11	4	84	0.28	0.10	8
0.04	9	4	69	0.10	0.06	5
0.43	5	18	300	31	4.50	162
0.05	1.34	2.86	63	4	0.54	150
0	102	0	111	0	0	415
0.10	43	22	295	0	4	231
0.04	11	18	403	1.24	0.16	61
0.10	301	27	406	5	1	83
0	80	60	440	3	0.90	100
0.47	32	9	70	6	0.30	158
0.10	5	10	355	8	0.70	15
0	311	63	196	18	2	296
1	8	12	273	0	0.23	70
0.26	19	51	175	0	1.43	150
0.14	7	0.30	0.67	0.08	0	10
0.39	86	19	152	3	0.41	370
0.12	6	7	22	9	13	41
0.65	96	15	133	10	0.30	173
1.40	41	13	207	11	0.66	216
0.70	6	9	186	0.10	0.17	70
0	12	51	214	2	1	190
2	15	50	186	2	1	165

	VITAMIN A (MCG)	VITAMIN B₁ (THIAMIN) (MG)	VITAMIN B₆ (MG)	FOLATE (MCG)	VITAMIN ((MG)
RDAS FOR MEN/WOMEN	**900/700**	**1.2/1.1**	**1.3/1.3**	**400/400**	**90/75**
Pear (1 medium)	1.60	0.02	0.05	12	7
Pepper, chile, raw (½ pepper)	21.6	0.03	0.23	10.35	65
Peppers, sweet (10 strips)	78	0.04	0.13	13	70
Pie, apple (1 piece)	37	0.03	0.04	32	4
Pizza, cheese (1 slice)	74	0.20	0.04	35	1
Pizza, vegetable (1 slice)	58	0.40	0.50	116	79
Plum (1)	21	0.03	0.05	1.45	6
Popcorn (1 cup)	0.80	0.02	0.02	2	0
Pork (3 ounces)	0	0.80	0.30	3	0
Potatoes, mashed (1 cup)	8.40	0.20	0.50	17	13
Potato salad (1 cup)	2.93	0.20	0.40	19	19
Potpie, chicken	256	0.30	0.20	41	2
Pretzels (10 twists)	0	0.30	0.07	103	0
Raisins (1.5 ounces)	0	0.05	0.08	1.28	2.30
Raspberries (10)	0.38	0.01	0.01	4	5
Rice, brown (1 cup)	0	0.20	0.30	8	0
Rice, white (1 cup)	0	0.03	0.15	5	0
Ricotta cheese, part skim (½ cup)	132	0.03	0.02	16	0
Salad dressing, light Italian (1 tablespoon)	0	0	0	0	0
Salmon (3 ounces)	9.84	0.20	0.71	22	0
Salsa (½ cup)	44	0.05	0.16	21	18
Sauerkraut (1 cup)	1.42	0.03	0.18	34	21
Sausage (1 link)	0	0.05	0.01	0.26	0
Shrimp (4 large)	0	0.01	0.03	0.77	0.48
Soft drink with caffeine (12 ounces)	0	0	0	0	0
Soup, cream of chicken (1 cup)	179	0.07	0.07	7	1.24

VITAMIN E (MG)	CALCIUM (MG)	MAGNESIUM (MG)	POTASSIUM (MG)	SELENIUM (MCG)	ZINC (MG)	CALORIES
15/15	1,000/1,000	420/320	3500/3500	55/55	11/8	
0.20	15	12	198	0.17	0.17	100
0.30	6	10	145	0.20	0.12	2
0.36	7	6.46	105	0	0	5
1.78	13	8	76	1	0.20	296
0	117	16	113	13	1	272
2	189	65	548	23	2	170
0	3	5	114	0.30	0.07	40
0	1	11	24	0.80	0.30	31
0.20	6	15	253	14	2	191
0.04	46	38	621	2	0.60	201
0.14	14	36	551	10	0.60	358
4	33	24	256	0.70	1	484
0.21	22	21	88	3	0.50	229
0.30	12	13	350	0.26	0.08	127
0.17	5	4	28	0.04	0.08	10
0.06	20	84	84	19	1	216
0.06	16	19	55	12	0.80	205
0.09	337	19	155	21	1.70	171
0	0	0	2	0.20	0	26
0.95	11	28	475	35	0.60	175
1.53	39	17	275	0.50	0.30	41
0.14	43	18	241	0.90	0.30	45
0.03	1.30	1.56	25	1.87	0.24	125
0	9	7	40	9	0.30	22
0	10	3	3	0.34	0	154
0.25	181	17	272	8	0.67	225

	VITAMIN A (MCG)	VITAMIN B₁ (THIAMIN) (MG)	VITAMIN B₆ (MG)	FOLATE (MCG)	VITAMIN C (MG)
RDAS FOR MEN/WOMEN	**900/700**	**1.2/1.1**	**1.3/1.3**	**400/400**	**90/75**
Soup, tomato (1 cup)	29.28	0.09	0.11	15	66
Soybeans (1 cup cooked)	14	0.47	0.10	200	31
Spaghetti with meatballs (1½ cups)	46	0.38	0.43	101	24
Spareribs (3 ounces)	1.91	0.26	0.22	3	0
Spinach (1 cup)	140	0.02	0.06	58	8
Steak (different cuts)	0	0.10	0.30	6	0
Strawberries (1 cup)	1.66	0.03	0.09	40	97
Submarine sandwich	71	1	0.10	87	12
Sunflower seeds (¼ cup)	5	0	0.28	82	0.50
Sweet potato (1)	350	0.09	0.25	9	19
Taco salad (1.5 cups)	71	0.10	0.20	83	4
Toaster pastry (1)	148	0.20	0.20	15	0
Tofu (4 ounces)	4.96	0.10	0.06	19	0
Tomato (1 medium)	26	0.02	0.05	9	8
Tuna salad (1 cup)	49	0.06	0.17	16	5
Turkey, skinless (½ breast)	0	0.16	2.26	31	0
Vegetable juice (1 cup)	188	0.10	0.30	51	67
Walnuts (1 cup)	37	0.27	0.70	82	4
Watermelon (1 wedge)	104	0.20	0.40	6	31
Wheat germ (½ cup)	0	0.20	0.40	81	0
Whey protein powder (2 teaspoons)	0	0	0	0	0
Wine, red (3.5 ounces)	0	0	0.03	2	0
Wine, white (3.5 ounces)	0	0	0.01	0	0
Yogurt, low-fat (8 ounces)	2	0.10	0.09	24	1.70

VITAMIN E (MG)	CALCIUM (MG)	MAGNESIUM (MG)	POTASSIUM (MG)	SELENIUM (MCG)	ZINC (MG)	CALORIES
15/15	**1,000/1,000**	**420/320**	**3500/3500**	**55/55**	**11/8**	
2	12	7	263	0.50	0.24	180
0.02	261	108	970	3	1.64	298
4	138	66	718	39	5	545
0.20	30	15	204	24	3	338
0.60	30	24	167	0.30	0.16	10
0.11	4	19	250	12	3.26	217
0.50	27	22	253	1	0.20	46
0	189	68	394	31	2.60	386
12	42	127	248	21.42	1.82	205
1.42	41	27	348	0.30	0.30	103
192	51	416	4	3	0	279
0.90	17	12	57	6.30	0.30	204
0.01	434	37	150	11	1	75
0.33	6	7	146	0	0.11	35
2	35	39	365	84	1	383
0.30	39	109	1,142	95	5	413
12	26	27	467	1	0.50	50
0	73	253	655	21	4.28	654
0.40	41	31	479	0.30	0.20	86
0	27	275	166	91	14	104
0	0	0	260	0	0	21
0	8	13	111	0.20	0.10	88
0	9	10	80	0.20	0.07	86
0	415	37	497	11	1.88	193

GLYCEMIC LOADS FOR SELECTED FOODS

Peanuts	1	All-Bran cereal	9
Low-fat yogurt, artificially sweetened	2	Grapefruit juice	9
		Hamburger bun	9
Carrots	3	Kidney beans, canned	9
Grapefruit	3	Lentil soup	9
Green peas	3	Oatmeal cookies	9
Fat-free milk	4	Sweet corn	9
Pear	4	American rye bread	10
Watermelon	4	Cheese tortellini	10
Beets	5	Frozen waffles	10
Orange	5	Honey	10
Peach	5	Lima beans, frozen	10
Plum	5	Low-fat yogurt, sweetened with sugar	10
Apple	6	Pinto beans	10
Kiwifruit	6	White bread	10
Tomato soup	6	Bran Chex cereal	11
Baked beans	7	Apple juice	12
Chickpeas, canned	7	Banana	12
Grapes	7	Kaiser roll	12
Pineapple	7	Orange juice	12
Whole-wheat bread	7	Saltine crackers	12
Popcorn	8	Bran flakes	13
Soy milk	8	Oatmeal	13
Taco shells	8		

Graham crackers	14	Total cereal	17
Special K cereal	14	Brown rice	18
Vanilla wafers	14	Fettuccine	18
Bran muffin	15	Angel food cake	19
Cheerios cereal	15	Cornflakes cereal	21
French bread	15	French fries	22
Grape-Nuts cereal	15	Jelly beans	22
Mashed potatoes	15	Macaroni	22
Shredded wheat cereal	15	Rice Krispies cereal	22
Bread stuffing mix	16	Couscous	23
Cheese pizza	16	Linguine	23
Whole-wheat spaghetti	16	Long-grain rice	23
Black bean soup	17	White rice	23
Blueberry muffin	17	Bagel	25
Corn chips	17	Baked potato	26
Doughnut	17	Spaghetti	27
Grape-Nuts Flakes cereal	17	Raisins	28
Instant oatmeal	17	Macaroni and cheese	32
Rice cakes	17	Instant rice	36
Sweet potato	17		

How to Use This Chart

The numbers in this chart represent the glycemic loads (GLs) of common foods. The GL is the product of a food's glycemic index and the amount of carbohydrates available per serving. Essentially, the GL estimates the projected elevation in blood glucose caused by eating a particular food. The higher a food's GL, the higher it is likely to be in both calories and carbs, so try to center your meals around foods with a GL of 19 or less and shoot for a total GL of less than 120 for the whole day.

INDEX

Boldface page references indicate photographs.
Underscored references indicate boxed text.

A

D

Insulin, 12, 13, <u>54</u>, 63, <u>68</u>, 82, 114, 122
Insulin resistance, <u>54</u>, <u>55</u>, 63
Intensity, 10–11, 172–73
Internal oblique muscles, <u>212</u>
Interval training
    cardiovascular exercise, <u>172</u>, 173, 175
    fat burned by, 206
    high-intensity cycling, 173
    workouts
        15-Minute Rope Burn, 209
        The Pyramid, 206, 209
        20-Minute Sprinter, 206
Irritable bowel syndrome, improving with exercise, 10
Isothiocyanates, <u>105</u>

J

Jogging, 44
Joint pain, 20–21
Jumping rope, 209
Junk food, 15, 121

K

Kidney beans, <u>102</u>, 152
Kidney disease, <u>4</u>, <u>23</u>
Kneeling three-way cable crunch, 261, **261**
Knee raise
    bent-leg, 225, **225**
    with drop, 267, **267**
    hanging, 227, **227**
    hanging single-knee, 260, **260**
    Swiss ball, 232, **232**
Knee raise with drop, 267, **267**

L

Lactic acid, <u>172</u>
Lateral medicine ball blast, 266, **266**
LDL cholesterol, <u>38–41</u>, 57
Leg curl, 200–201, **200–201**
Leg-extension, 196, **196**
Leg soreness, <u>172</u>
Legumes, 103–4
Lentils, <u>103</u>
Leptin, <u>20</u>, 110, 122

Licorice, <u>25</u>
Lima beans, <u>24</u>
Linea alba, 271
Lipoproteins, <u>38</u>, 58, 124
Long-arm weighted crunch, 221, **221**
Longevity, increase with
    flat belly, 13–15
    nuts, 9
    raw vegetables, 8
Lower back, exercises for
    back extension, 249, **249**
    swimmer's backstroke, 252, **252**
    Swiss ball superman, 251, **251**
    twisting back extension, 250, **250**
Lunch recipes, 139–45
    Guac and Roll, 141
    Guilt-Free BLT, 141
    Hot Tuna, 142
    Hurry Curry, 144
    The I-Am-Not-Eating-Salad Salad, 140
    The Johnny Apple Cheese Sandwich, 139
    The Melon Banquet, 145
    Nice-to-Meat-You Sandwich, 143
    Popeye and Olive Oil, 144
    The Two Chicks, 145
    Yo Soup for You, 143
Lunge, traveling, 202–3, **202–3**
Lutein, <u>24</u>, <u>41</u>, <u>105</u>
Lycopene, <u>24</u>, <u>74–75</u>
Lying cable crunch, 219, **219**

M

Macular degeneration, <u>105</u>
Magnesium
    benefits of, <u>25</u>, 100, 101
    in common foods, <u>287</u>, <u>289</u>, <u>291</u>, <u>293</u>, <u>295</u>, <u>297</u>
    sources of, <u>25</u>, 101, <u>105</u>
Mandarin oranges, 144
Meal plan (7-day), <u>94–95</u>
Meal replacement bars, 85
Meals
    apportionment of calories, <u>12</u>
    cheat meal, 96–97
    eating out, <u>142</u>
    number of, 32, 88–89
    planning for next day, 33
    portion control, <u>6</u>, 92–93